The Evolution
of
Pre-hospital
Emergency Care

Belfast and Beyond

The Evolution of Pre-hospital Emergency Care

Belfast and Beyond

John S. Geddes

MB BCh BAO (The Queen's University of Belfast)
BSc, MD, FRCP (Lond), FACC
Consultant Cardiologist, Royal Victoria Hospital, Belfast
(1971-1987)
Associate Professor of Medicine, University of Manitoba
(1987-1999)

Ronald D. Stewart

MD (Dalhousie University)
OC, ONS, BA, BSc, FACEP, DSc (Hon), LLD(Hon)
Professor Emeritus, Medical Education,
Professor of Emergency Medicine, Dalhousie University, Halifax, Nova Scotia
Adjunct Professor of Emergency Medicine,
University of Pittsburgh
Adjunct Professor, Cape Breton University, Nova Scotia

Thomas F. Baskett

MB BCh BAO (The Queen's University of Belfast)
FRCS(C), FRCS (Ed), FRCOG, FACOG, DHMSA
Professor Emeritus, Obstetrics and Gynaecology
Dalhousie University, Halifax, Nova Scotia

Clinical Press 2017

On Emergency Care

"Success in the recovery of the apparently dead, is related to the length of time that elapses before the proper remedies can be applied."

Charles Kite
An Essay on the Recovery of the Apparently Drowned. London; C. Dilly: 1788

"The more the danger is great and pressing, the more the response must be prompt and energetic."

Dominique-Jean Larrey
Mémoires de chirurgie militaire, et compagnes.
Paris: J. Smith (1812-1817) Vol11

"Death in hearts too good to die"

Claude Beck
JAMA 1960;174:118

"The human suffering and financial loss from preventable accidental death constitute a public health problem second only to the ravages of ancient plagues or world wars."

Accidental Death and Disability: the Neglected Disease of Modern Society
National Academy of Sciences-National Research Council, Washington,
DC 1966.

"The majority of deaths ascribed to coronary artery disease occur outside hospital. Those who are admitted to hospital represent, in fact, the survivors of a storm which has already taken its main toll."

RH McNeilly and J Pemberton
BMJ 1968;3:142

"Well if that is so .....We must go out and get these people."

Frank Pantridge 1965

"History written by participants is personal. That makes it more lively, but also inevitably biased. We all stand on the shoulders of those before us. What ultimately counts is that progress was made, not who gets the credit."

Peter Safar, *Bull Anesth Hist 2001;19:1.*

While the advice and information in this book is believed to be true and accurate at the time of going to press, neither the authors, the editors, nor the publisher can accept legal responsibility for any errors of omissions that may be made. The publisher makes no warranty, express or implied, with respect to the material conatined herein

Published by: Clinical Press Ltd., Redland Green Farm, Redland, Bristol, BS6 7HF, UK.

British Library Cataloguing in Publication Data

Geddes John S., Stewart Ronald D., Baskett, Thomas F.
Evolution of Pre-hospital Emergency Care, Belfast and beyond

1. Pre-Hospital **Emergency Care, Evolution of**

ISBN 978-1-85457-093-2

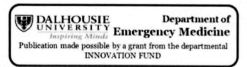

DALHOUSIE **Department of**
UNIVERSITY **Emergency Medicine**
Inspiring Minds
Publication made possible by a grant from the departmental
INNOVATION FUND

Contents

Foreword

Pre-hospital emergency care is an expectation of life in developed countries. But this was not always the case and in fact the birth and subsequent evolution to achieve rapidly provided, high quality care occurred only 50 years ago. For such a vital safety net in our lives it is gratifying to read Geddes, Stewart, and Baskett's account of the birth and early development of such an important public service.

Among the myriad medical emergencies treated by pre-hospital emergency care, the most important is resuscitation from sudden cardiac arrest. Sudden cardiac arrest was uniformly and universally fatal until 1967 when Frank Pantridge and John Geddes (yes, the co-author of this book) in Belfast, Northern Ireland published the results of a landmark programme. Their innovation brought care directly to the patient with a mobile intensive care unit and demonstrated that resuscitation with defibrillation and advanced medical care could save lives outside hospitals. This book is aptly named "From Belfast and Beyond" because from the first programme came an explosion of similar and variant programmes spreading first to the United States and then throughout the world.

This book celebrates the origins and early development of out of hospital resuscitative care. There is much to celebrate. Consider the accomplishments of the past 50 years: resuscitation, particularly from ventricular fibrillation, is commonplace. The science of resuscitation is well defined. Effective training programmes for basic and advanced skills are in place. Automated external defibrillators (AEDs) allow first responders and the general public to provide defibrillation quickly. Public training in CPR and use of AEDs are widespread. Many emergency dispatch centres provide telephone CPR. Mandatory CPR training is required in high schools in many states and countries. Automatic alerting of volunteers to nearby cardiac arrests can shorten the time to care.

These accomplishments are worth celebrating but considerably more needs to be done. Overall survival from ventricular fibrillation remains low. Perhaps most disappointing is the wide disparity in survival. While some communities can achieve survival of over 50% most cannot, and furthermore the disparity among communities is five-fold or greater. It is a sad reality that the city in which the cardiac arrest occurs is a major determinant of survival. The challenge is to understand the impediments to high performance and to implement and disseminate programmes proven to increase survival.

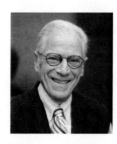

So while we will never stop working to achieve the promise of quality resuscitation in all communities, let us pause to toast Pantridge and Geddes and the pioneers who followed to make resuscitation a reality and daily snatch life from the jaws of death.

Mickey Eisenberg MD PhD
Professor of Emergency Medicine, University of Washington
Director, Medical QI, King County Emergency Medical Services

Preface

The year 2017 marks the 50th anniversary of the landmark paper by Pantridge and Geddes, describing the organisation and results of the first hospital-based mobile coronary care ambulance at the Royal Victoria Hospital, Belfast, Northern Ireland. The 'cardiac ambulance' was started on 1st January 1966, and the report in the 5th August 1967 edition of the Lancet recorded the first fifteen months' experience.

This book covers the early development of mobile coronary care within the context of major societal and scientific changes leading to emergency intensive care, cardio-pulmonary resuscitation and defibrillation. The success of the cardiac ambulance stimulated the development of broader pre-hospital emergency services and the concomitant growth of associated areas of expertise and paramedical personnel.

A second rationale for publishing this book now is to have it coincide with the October, 2017 meeting in Halifax, Nova Scotia celebrating both the 50th anniversary of mobile coronary care and the 20th anniversary of the Nova Scotia emergency health services system.

The three authors of this book: John Geddes (JSG), Tom Baskett (TFB) and Ronald Stewart (RDS) all have links to the background and development of pre-hospital emergency care.

JSG was the co-founder, together with Frank Pantridge, of mobile coronary care, and his seminal role is outlined in various chapters of this book. In particular, he was uniquely placed and involved in the first 20 years of the Belfast experience.

TFB grew up in the same village, Hillsborough, Co Down, as Frank Pantridge. During the years 1963-65, he served as a clinical clerk and house physician on Dr Pantridge's unit. In the late 1960s he went out regularly with the Belfast obstetric flying squad ambulance – the counterpart of the cardiac ambulance. Subsequently he was involved for many years with the provision of emergency obstetric care to remote areas of the Canadian north.

RDS began as a general practitioner in the north Highlands on Nova Scotia's Cape Breton Island, later becoming one of the first residents in Emergency Medicine at Los Angeles County/USC Medical Centre – the first emergency medicine academic department in the world. In his subsequent position as the first Medical Director of the Paramedic Programme in Los Angeles County he met up with Frank Pantridge at many meetings in the United States, the UK and Europe. He later became Medical Director of the Pittsburgh EMS system and founded the Center for Emergency Medicine at the University of Pittsburgh, now the largest Emergency Medicine research and education institute in the country. Upon return to his home province of Nova Scotia he was elected to the provincial parliament and became Minister of Health, in which role he established a province-wide EMS system with regionalised trauma care, ground and aeromedical critical care transport, a research foundation, and a broadening of paramedical curricula and scope of practice.

Acknowledgements

The source of the following illustrations is acknowledged with gratitude:

- Figures 1.2, 2.3 and 2.4 The Safar Collection, University of Pittsburgh;
- Figure 1.4 Nova Scotia Archives;
- Figures 3.2 and 11.5 John Geddes;
- Figures 3.3 and 4.5 Elsevier Publishing;
- Figures 4.2 and front cover John Geddes (photo by George Craig),
- 4.3 and 4.4 John Geddes (photos by Peter Williamson);
- Figure 6.1 Library of Congress Prints and Photographs Division. Look Magazine Collection;
- Figure 6.2 Eugene Nagel;
- Figures 6.3 Leonard Cobb;
- Figure 6.4 Richard Crampton;
- Figure 7.1 Pantridge Trust;
- Figure 7.2 Casino Nova Scotia (Sydney);
- Figures 10.1 to 10.10 Supplied by Emergency Medical Care, Inc and the Department of Emergency Medicine, Division of EMS, Dalhousie University;
- Figures 11.1 and 11.4 Elizabeth Pantridge;
- Figures 11.6 and 11.7 Tom Baskett.

The remaining figures are from the quoted reference or in the public domain.

RDS wishes to acknowledge the contribution of Dr. Brian Zink and his ongoing work in compiling a history of the specialty of Emergency Medicine in his book, *Anyone, Anything, Anytime: A History of Emergency Medicine*.

Chapter 1

The stage is set

Discoveries are made when the time for making them is ripe, and not before; the stage is set, the time is ripe, and the event occurs...[1]

If there was a 'eureka moment' in the history of emergency medical services (EMS) it was inconspicuous, and its importance was not realised until much later. In our account we will hear how, in the autumn of 1956, during an automobile ride somewhere between Kansas City and Chicago, two clinician-scientists fresh from a national conference of the emerging specialty of anaesthesia realised they had more in common than they thought. They were both interested in saving lives by investigating various methods of rescue breathing. Drs. Jim Elam and Peter Safar had a growing interest in resuscitation which would result in the saving of thousands- if not millions- of lives. And the 'starting gun' for the search that would eventually result in what we now know as cardio-pulmonary resuscitation (CPR) came about as a result of the meeting of these two great minds. They discussed pooling their ideas and resources in an effort to prove mouth-to-mouth breathing was far superior to the manual methods taught and used by various agencies and health professionals of the day. Before the trip ended the two informally agreed to pursue further research into:

1. relief of airway obstruction by the tissues of the neck and pharynx by jaw-lift and extension of the head;
2. air volumes delivered via manual versus mouth-to-mouth ventilation techniques; and
3. the feasibility of direct mouth-to-mouth ventilation without the use of adjunct devices.[2] (Figures 1.1 and 1.2)

The humble beginnings of emergency resuscitation research resulted from that cross-country journey, and the results of those humble beginnings shook the world. But they were not alone in their belief that medical care could and must be improved for those fellow-humans who, often through no fault of their own, risked losing life or limb.

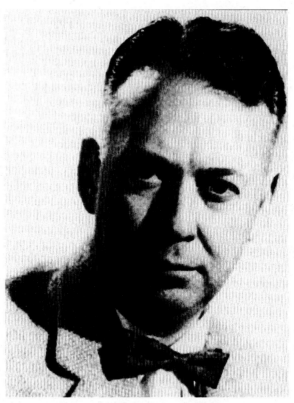

Figure 1.1 James Otis Elam (1918-1995). As research anaesthetist in St Louis, Missouri he demonstrated that exhaled air was adequate for artificial ventilation, which underpinned the development of modern CPR.

Their sometimes-daring approach to solving the problem of such emergency situations was reflected less than a decade later in the equally daring idea put into practice by Drs. Pantridge and Geddes in Belfast. These two pioneers acted on their logical but seemingly outlandish idea of taking medical care out of the confines of the hospital- in that case the coronary care unit- directly to the location where people were stricken. They reasoned, if most of the deaths occurred within an hour or two after the onset of the victims' heart attacks, who could not therefore receive potentially life-saving treatment, why not reach them as soon as possible so that death might be avoided, either by preventing ventricular fibrillation or by appropriate first aid followed by a timely electric shock – proven to be effective several years earlier? In the development of emergency care for those at risk, this idea- extending the treatment and technology outside the walls of the hospital- was, for those of us in medicine, our version of a eureka moment, and our medical world was, indeed, never again to be the same.[3]

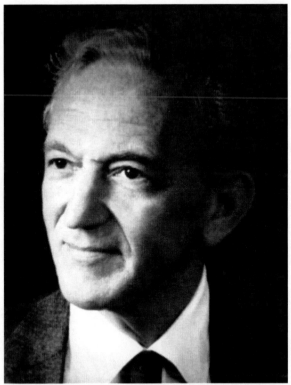

Figure 1.2 Peter Safar (1924-2003). While working as an anaesthetist in Baltimore he promoted the simple head tilt and chin lift method to overcome airway obstruction in the unconscious patient. His prodigious and sustained research over many years in Baltimore and Pittsburgh contributed much to the evolution of CPR.

The time is ripe

As with most events in history, these and other opportunities seldom happen purely by chance. Most breakthroughs are the result of a wonderful mixture of unpredictable circumstances, seemingly unrelated phenomena, or just plain serendipity- or even stupidity. Or they may be the product of long years of hard work, and even then great discoveries may not be appreciated as such or can even be ignored when considered insignificant. Gradually, from the middle of the 20th to well into the 21st century events and circumstances have combined to offer better ways of treating illness, repairing the damage we humans cause to each other, or preventing illness and death. Many of these improvements and changes we have seen in the past fifty or more years have come about not as eureka moments at all, but rather as the result of events, circumstances and trends which, at the time, we might never have recognised as relevant, much less important.

Why, then, did the decade leading up to and including the sixties

3

influence so heavily the direction in which emergency care developed and improved and, to a degree at least, brought these benefits of medicine to the highways, byways, the hovels and the homes of so many communities? And so rapidly. To understand this phenomenon and how it occurred so relatively quickly we are obliged to pay close attention to the social, technological and medical developments of the fifties and sixties. Some are more easily understood and documented than others but the most important would include:

1. The post-war rise in standards of living in both Europe and North America.
2. Improvement in public health, nutrition, access to health care, and the resulting increased longevity.
3. Improvement in medical technology and diagnostics.
4. The rise of hospitals.
5. The trend toward physician specialisation.
6. The decline of the house call.
7. The rise of the automobile/mass transportation.
8. The flight to the suburbs.
9. The increasing influence of mass media, especially television.
10. Increasing government involvement in design/funding of health services.
11. The fallout from war.

Live long and prosper[*]

Despite the devastation wreaked upon humankind by World War II, economic recovery began within years of war's end in both Europe and North America. The Marshall Plan in Europe[4] and the economic and social changes which were occurring in both the United States and Canada resulted in a dramatic and rapid improvement in post-war standards of living. The expansion of the National Health Service in the United Kingdom was central to improvement in health care delivered to large population groups. And the introduction of unemployment insurance, national Medicare and Pension Plans, combined with welcoming immigration policies allowed even the huge, sparsely populated and young country of Canada to far exceed even its own aspirations. These changes heralded a new age of rapid improvement in the social determinants of health and consequently an increase in life expectancy, particularly in Canada, the Scandinavian countries and Western Europe.[5] The effect of medical technology and diagnostics on population health in the mid-20th century

---

A blessing from the Orthodox Jewish tradition
(used with a modified hand gesture by Leonard Nemoy as Mr. Spock in the Star Trek TV series)

mostly reflected the growing victory over infectious disease through immunisation, antisepsis, chemotherapeutic antibiotics and our increasing ability to identify new infectious agents. These advances allowed us to barely keep ahead of newer threats, some of which were visited upon us by the indiscriminate use of antibiotics. Despite that, progress was real; the eradication from the planet of the scourge of smallpox was announced in 1977 [6], and cases of poliomyelitis have declined from a mid-century incidence of almost 60,000 in the United States alone to a confirmed world-wide total of only thirty-two cases in 2004.[7]   Infectious diseases ceased to be the chief cause of death as the 20th century progressed.[8] By mid-century cardiovascular diseases had assumed first place, peaking at the end of the sixties, although age-adjusted rates were cut in half by the year 2000.[9] This remarkable decline began before the advent of resuscitation programmes or other medical interventions, so care should be taken not to assume a cause-and-effect relationship, although early evidence suggested it.[10-12] Our recounting of the early and current experience throughout the fifty years would support the opinion that lower death rates from cardiovascular disease is a result of many factors, of which early and aggressive interventions - rapid mobile intensive care, defibrillation, thrombolysis, etc.- are but a part.[12] But such interventions may be even more impressive as more data, particularly in relation to early thrombolysis, are gathered from modern emergency medical services systems, coronary treatment centres and research institutes .

Temples of Healing[+]

Throughout the 20th century, and particularly in the last half, health care became increasingly centred in hospitals. Citizens began to view the hospital no longer as the 19th century poor house or dying factory rank with filth and disease, but rather as a refuge designed to care and to cure. That gradual but profound change took almost a century, well after the cleansing battles waged by Florence Nightingale or the pungent odours of carbolic acid wafting through the wards of Mr. Lister and his disciples as they forever changed surgery. The advent of anaesthesia, along with 'Listerism' and its progression to aseptic surgery, permitted surgeons to rely more on their skill than their speed, while reducing the risk of sepsis and increasing the chances of patients surviving their ministrations. As evidence in the medical and surgical literature built a convincing case for asepsis in surgery and revealed the inherent dangers of inhaled anaesthetics,

---

+ Ancient 'Temples of Healing' were dedicated to the Greek god of healing and medicine, Asclepius, perhaps the ancestors of our modern hospitals.

physicians gradually began to concentrate more and more upon less and less. In other words, specialisation took hold and became the norm. This favoured an increase in sophistication of techniques and technology, the resulting expense requiring the concentration of equipment and specialists in the modern 'temples of healing'- hospitals.

The trend toward specialisation led inevitably to greater sophistication and an expansion of services offered by hospitals. Surgical intervention no longer represented, in the 20th century, a late effort to save a life or limb. Surgery expanded to include daring- but now routine- probing of the body's every nook and cranny; every organ, including the brain, was subject to surgical repair or manipulation. The increasing drama of medicine became an object of fascination on the part of the public. One of the most notable breakthroughs of modern medicine, the discovery and stellar success of the polio vaccine, was widely reported in the public press and Salk and his colleagues were seen as heroes in white coats[13]; their currency grew with the advent and huge popularity of the cinematic and television doctor.[14] Our account will later focus on the major role mass media can play in the public perception of, and attitude towards medicine, its practitioners and the results of their labour in the context of immediate care.[14,15] (see Chapter 8)

Research into new methods of treatment grew exponentially, leading surgeons and other specialists to attempt procedures and potions for conditions which, up to the post-war era, were largely considered hopeless or at least far too risky. Pushing the envelope led to the occasional disaster followed by a search for a management strategy for complications or untoward results. Early use of chloroform and ether, particularly when accompanied- for whatever reason- by hypoxia, could lead to ventricular irritability expressed as the disaster of ventricular fibrillation (VF). Reversing this disaster required the application of an electric current, in the early cases at least, directly to the heart. Surgeons seeking to repair cardiac defects would occasionally be faced with the unexpected catastrophe of fibrillation and protocols were developed following the first successful defibrillation of the heart of a fourteen-year-old boy by the American surgeon Claude Beck in 1947.[16] (Figure 1.3)

Such occurrences prompted more research into how best to resolve these events, and the answers were forthcoming within the decade, with widespread implications well beyond the laboratory or operating theatre.

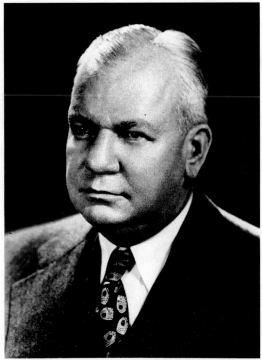

Cleander S. Beck

Figure 1.3 Claude Schaeffer Beck (1894-1971)A thoracic surgeon in Cleveland, Beck was the first to successfully correct ventricular fibrillation with a directly applied defibrillator to the heart. He also demonstrated that in many cases of fatal ventricular fibrillation, the post-mortem examination of the heart showed minimal disease and coined the phrase, 'hearts too good to die', to support active attempts at resuscitation in sudden cardiac arrest.

Knowing more and more…about less and less

The increasing recognition of hospitals by the public as centres of health care, if not temples of healing, was paralleled and fostered by the dramatic **expansion of physician specialisation**, especially in the United States. In 1938 the percentage of physicians self-designating as general practitioners was just over 79%; in 1970 that number had declined to just over 17% of clinicians in practice. Those identifying themselves as specialist increased from 21% in 1938, to over 75% of practicing clinicians in 1970.[17,18]

In both Europe and North America the **rise of physician specialisation** and the decrease in the number of general practitioners resulted in the **decline of the house call** as a medical tradition of general practice[19] (Figure 1.4) and forced citizens to hospital or clinics for their health care needs.[20]

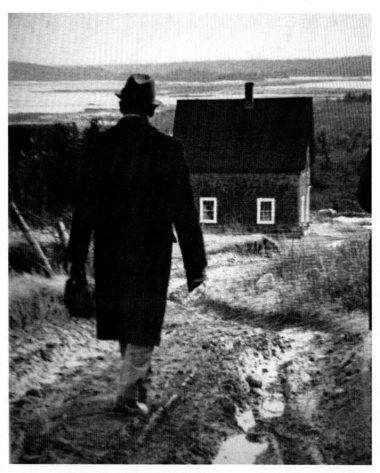

Figure 1.4 Physician house calls, especially in rural or under-serviced areas were time-consuming, inefficient and faded from the health care scene in the 60s-70s, putting pressure on hospitals to fill the need for primary care - particularly the emergency room.

This decline was less striking and slower to develop in Britain and Canada, in part due to cultural differences and public expectations but also because national health systems covered fees for home visits. In America private insurance plans encouraged a reduction in physician visits, culminating in the 1980s and onward in managed care by large corporate interests and the bureaucracy at its base.[21] The decrease in the number of general practitioners, combined with the greater number of hospital emergency facilities (if not in the quality of care they offered), led as well during the decade of the sixties to the perception of a health care system in crisis and forced a close examination of how citizens accessed medical care.[22] Physicians added to the overcrowding of emergency facilities by replacing the house call with *"I'll-see-you-in-the-emergency-room"* advice to patients.[23] Hospitals accommodated the rapid rise in specialisation and physician demands by providing proper tools and incentives for their work; the latest equipment, expanded roles in hospital governance and increasing pay levels. Most institutions, however, invested little in providing quality physician coverage of emergency departments and relied during the sixties on inexperienced house staff (interns and residents), contract physicians at any level of expertise, or the even less effective means of attempting to educate the public in the appropriate use of emergency facilities.[24] Without adequate policy safeguards, standards and methods of monitoring quality of care, these methods were doomed to fail, and served rather to expose hospitals to potential legal battles and public relations disasters.

Five additional societal trends added to the forces reshaping the delivery of emergency and primary health care in both Europe and North America: **the rise of the automobile** and increasing mobility of the population, **the flight to the suburbs** from the inner cities, particularly of the United States, **the increasing influence of mass media**, and **the growing involvement of government in funding and planning of health services**. Influencing all of these elements were **non-governmental agencies, associations and interest groups** targeting aspects of health and medicine: organ associations (e.g. heart, lung, liver groups), life-saving societies, and public health coalitions. As populations relocated out of the cities to the suburbs and migration of families was made easier with the family automobile, connections to health care services loosened, adding to the reduction of ties to private generalist physicians.

As the economy recovered and the standard of living for families in both North America and Europe improved after World War II, the automobile was king. Sales soared, and as the second half of the 20th century progressed, the recovery of the Japanese economy soon outpaced the rise in Europe and America.[25] As noted already, populations became mobile, construction of major highways served the boom in auto sales and liberated families in a way never before seen; the result, sadly, saw carnage on the roads which quickly became recognised as a public health burden and one of the greatest killers of the young.[26] If one judges by health budgets invested in either programmes of prevention or research monies, the conclusion can be drawn that the population, until relatively recently, ascribed the toll of disability and death to an inevitable result of progress or acts of the Almighty. But change was to come in the sixties through a report which, coupled with the turmoil in hospital emergency departments and the almost non-existent ambulance care in the streets and on the highways, led to a massive increase in attention to and funding from government to address the neglected disease of modern society- trauma.[27]

Playing doctor

The public was ready for, and slowly demanded, some answers; interest in health issues and medicine grew, aided by developing information technology. **The growing influence of mass media** - particularly television - provided organised Medicine with the tools to reach vast groups of people with a variety of health-related messages as well as ensuring that Hollywood and TV moguls could blunt the impact of falling revenues from declining cinema attendance.[28] The loosening of ties to general practitioners resulted from the growing trend towards physician specialisation, providing primary care in hospital emergency departments, and from the mobility of families. The increasing familiarity of the public with hospitals and their emergency services not only accustomed citizens to the ready availability of round-the-clock medical care but also, paradoxically, introduced them to the perceived and real defects of that care offered in crowded, tension-ridden, and the at-times unwelcoming environment of the often-overwhelmed emergency room - some blaming physicians, in general, for apathy and active self-interest.[29] Hospital boards and professional associations were well aware of the PR disasters looming as media and community activists soon began to agitate for improvements. After all, it was the decade of disruption- the Sixties- with all that implied.

With the advent of the cinematic representation of the 'good doctor' on the silver screen in the 1930s, the public, both in the United States and around the world, was introduced to a frequently idealised depiction of medicine and its practitioners. Such a portrait, whether accurate or not, was determined mostly by the general respect and admiration of the profession garnered by significant scientific breakthroughs as the mid-century approached. But in prewar Britain and America, movies helped by portraying physicians and organised medicine uniformly as heroic if not saintly, aided in this by boards of censors in both Europe and America. In fact, The British Board of Film Censors' rules clearly drew a protective curtain around a broad range of public figures and certain professions, outlined in their rules and regulations:[30]

"Incidents which bring into contempt public characters acting in their capacity as such, i.e., officers and men wearing His Majesty's Uniform, Ministers of Religion, Ministers of the Crown, Ambassadors and Representatives of Foreign Nations, Administrators of the Law, Medical Men, etc."[31]

And so there was an attempt to protect doctors from being cast in a bad, or even slightly shady, light. And in America, their own American Medical Association (AMA) kept a watchful eye in the guise of a twelve-man

Committee on Television, Radio and Motion Pictures formed in 1956. According to the enthusiastic journal article in the AMA's publication announcing this formal liaison between Hollywood and the healers, this committee was designed to help writers, producers or anyone else who might be striving for authenticity in their storylines:

"This spirit of cooperation between the medical profession and the television industry…is helping arouse today's mammoth public appetite for television shows with a medical flavor. Just so long as the menu includes authenticity with the basic story ingredients of action and suspense, the diet will be balanced for good health." [32]

This strategy was not new. In 1954 the originator of the early series *Medic* and NBC executives struck a tight deal with the Los Angeles County Medical Association which gave the low-budget drama access to ready-made (and therefore cheap) sets - the operating theatres and other facilities of the Los Angeles County Hospital. In return NBC was obliged to submit scripts for close examination to a twenty-man committee of this branch of the AMA - an arrangement which quickly foundered on the rocks of the constraints of television production deadlines.[33] Although the initial intention of the physician groups may well have been ensuring accuracy of medical procedures and disease/cure timelines, it soon became clear that the *approach* taken by script writers and directors could reflect well or not-so-well, on physicians, and on medicine or how it was practiced. Even in America, memory was raw in AMA circles of *The Citadel*, the 1938 British film clearly seen to favour the argument for a national health service (NHS) in the Britain of the late 1930s. It may have influenced, after its re-release in 1946 just prior to the introduction of NHS legislation, the parliamentary vote in favour of socialised medicine - the anathema of the AMA.[34]

The Sixties was the decade which saw a combination of large-scale print media with the developing technology of radio and television, which had major implications for health systems and rapid information exchange around the globe. Not only could scientists and clinicians more readily share ideas and the results of their research, but the public could hear or read the news of breakthroughs from scientific and medical sources, and from mass media- newspapers, radio, television and even magazines. Even now, fifty years on, we take note that less than twenty-six days after the publication of the *Lancet's* report of the success of the Belfast cardiac flying squad, *Time* magazine reported, accompanied by a photo of the mobile coronary care unit, the results of the Belfast breakthrough.[35]

Pounds, dollars and sense

The booming economy of the sixties provided fertile ground for innovations in health care delivery and **increasing government involvement in health system funding**; expenditures for American health care ballooned between 1950 and 1970 from $12.7 billion to $71.6 billion. Hospital renovation and expansion were boosted to the tune of $3.7 billion and, in response to complaints from the public and carping from clinicians, hospitals were forced to expand and ultimately, but not immediately, improve their emergency services.[36,37] By 1965 Federal legislation in the United States provided health insurance in the form of Medicare and Medicaid programmes for low-income earners, older citizens and people with disabilities.[38] Britain's National Health Service plan covered all citizens and was instituted country-wide in 1948,[39] and Canada's universal healthcare system was in place by 1968.[40]

By 1969 U.S. federal tax law required community hospitals, in order to retain their tax-exempt status, to provide 24-hour emergency services available to every citizen without regard to their ability to pay.[41] Many government and private insurance plans covered patients' visits to the emergency facility of a hospital, but not to private medical offices.[42] As could be expected, this encouraged citizens to present to emergency departments at any hour of the day or night, whenever they felt the need for medical advice or immediate care. And so visits to emergency departments exploded after 1950, the numbers augmented by hospital PR programmes which sold the fact that they offered round-the-clock care. So successful were these campaigns that emergency rooms became, essentially, community health centres. But many had very little capability of handling life-threatening emergencies and were often staffed by junior house officers (residents), contract physicians untrained for serious medical challenges, or even by inexperienced nurses, especially in off-hours.[43] This too was not new; as early as 1960 a survey conducted by the American College of Surgeons revealed major deficiencies in emergency departments across the United States,[44] setting the tone and the foundation for a major white paper some five years later which changed the course of emergency care across America and reaching well beyond. (see Chapter 8)

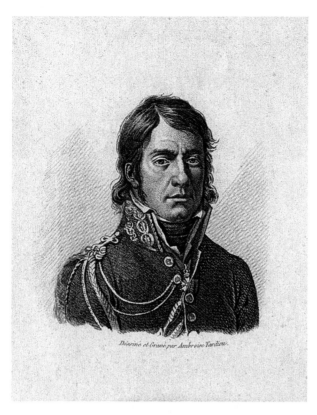

Figure 1.5
Dominique-Jean Larrey (1766-1842), Surgeon-in-Chief to the French Army of Napoleon Bonaparte, revolutionised the care of the injured soldier. He sent his medical teams to the wounded in the field of battle and was the first to apply a system of triage to their care.

The influence of war

To say that military medicine influenced for the better both clinical medicine and medical research is understating the major impact of the experience of war, from at least World War I to the present. But in our discussion of the evolution of emergency services, the brilliance of Dominique-Jean Larrey, Napoleon's chief surgeon, stands out in the history of immediate care of the wounded in the late 18th century.(Fig 1.5)

He conceived of using mobile teams of surgeons and assistants – 'ambulances volante'- with standard equipment and protocols and sending them to the wounded on the battlefield; rather than keeping them in stationary posts behind the lines to which injured soldiers would be taken.

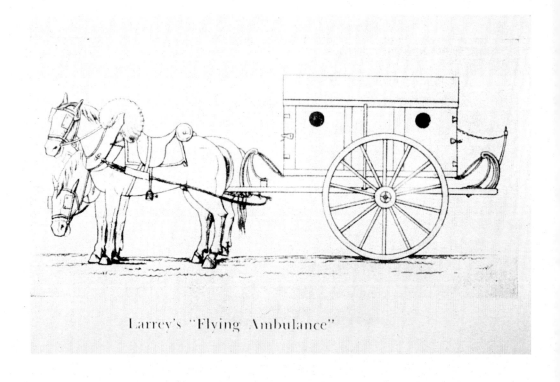

Larrey's "Flying Ambulance"

Figure 1.6
Larrey's 'Ambulance Volante' (flying ambulance) designed to take immediate care to wounded soldiers at the site of battle, and later redesigned to transport them back behind lines for more sophisticated treatment.

Larrey even designed sturdy carts which carried the equipment and personnel, later constructing them to carry the wounded as well.[45] (Figure 1.6)

Larrey adopted a method of sorting the wounded according to severity, which was refined in World War I and named by the French as *triage* [3]. This system of casualty care, upon which current regionalised trauma systems are designed, held as a governing principle the sorting of casualties and assigning each to a different level of care based on objective and pre-determined criteria.[46] But amid the atmosphere of rapid change in civilian trauma care in the sixties and onward, the governing influence was the experience of military medicine from World War II, and especially from the two more recent conflicts in Korea and Vietnam. Not only did the lessons from these two wars improve the clinical care of the wounded,[47] the organised system of triage and the importance of efficient and rapid transportation following appropriate, and sometimes high-level, field care were embedded in the minds of the medical teams who served. Many of them, on returning home to the United States, began to agitate for improvement of trauma care on the highways and byways as well as in the inner cities in which many of the academic medical centres were located.[48]

It was the Korean conflict which influenced most both the commissioning and the content of the report which changed the landscape of trauma care in the United States. The report was born of the desire of several surgeons who had served in Korea[49] and who, after demobilisation urged close scrutiny of the state of trauma care in America, the resulting report having the arresting title, *Accidental Death and Disability: The Neglected Disease of Modern Society,*[50] and the work of decades began.

The time is ripe...the stage is set

The decade of the Sixties is remembered for social change, rapid technological advancements born of research as well as serendipitous discoveries, increasing longevity in most population groups in the West, the beginning of the end of a divisive and brutal war in Southeast Asia and humans reaching towards the heavens and landing on the moon. Within the realm of health care, modern discoveries pushed the barriers of medicine and surgery beyond the dreams of most of us, citizens saw their entertainment thirst for the drama of medicine and health care slaked by film and television, and the mobility of people changed how we accessed care. Leaders in the field stepped up, took measured risks and broke through barriers to provide improved care and extended it to the streets, highways and even homes. The ingredients for discovery and innovation were there. The time was ripe...the stage was set. Enter the players....

References

1. Davidson CJ. quoted in Gaither's Dictionary of Scientific Quotations. Second ed., 2012, p. 540.
2. Safar P. From Vienna to Pittsburgh for Anesthesiology and Acute Medicine: An Autobiography. In: Careers in Anesthesiology: An Autobiographical Memoir. Fink BR, McGoldrick KE, editors. Park Ridge (IL): The Wood Library-Museum of Anesthesiology; 2000, p. 131.
3. Pantridge JF, Geddes JS: A mobile intensive care unit in the management of acute myocardial infarction. Lancet. 1967; 1:807-08.
4. United States Department of State, Bureau of Public Affairs. The Marshall Plan: Origins and Implementation. April 1967.

5. Palacios R: The future of global ageing. Int J Epidemiol 2002; 31:786-91.
6. Fenner F, Henderson DA, Arita I, Jezek Z, Ladnyi ID. Smallpox and its eradication. World Health Organization, Geneva, 1988.
7. Roberts L. Polio: the final assault? Science 2004; 303: 1961-68.
8. Jones DS, Podolsky SH, Greene JA. The burden of disease and the changing task of medicine. N Engl J Med 2012;366:2333-38.
9. Ford ES, Ajani UA, Croft JB, et al. Explaining the decrease in US deaths from coronary disease, 1980-2000. N Engl J Med 2007;356: 2388-98.
10. Crampton R, Aldrich RF, Gascho JA, Stillerman R. Reduction of prehospital, ambulance and coronary care death rates by the community-wide emergency cardiac care system. Am J Med 1975;58: 151-65.
11. Matthewson Z, McCloskey BG, Evans AE, Russell CJ, Wilson C. Mobile coronary care and community mortality from myocardial infarction. Lancet 1985; i:441-44.
12. Beaglehole R. Medical management and the decline in mortality from coronary artery disease. BMJ 1986;292:33-35.
13. Krieger J. "What price fame?" New York Times 1955; Magazine:Page 9.
14. Turow J. Playing doctor: television, storeytelling, and medical power. Ann Arbor: University of Michigan Press; 2010. p. 2.
15. Friedman LD. Introduction: through the looking glass: medical culture and the media. In: Friedman LD, editor. Cultural sutures: medicine and media. Durham, NC: Duke University Press; 2004. p.1-11.
16. Beck CS, Pritchard WH, Feil HS. Ventricular fibrillation of long duration abolished by electric shock. JAMA 1947;135:985-86.
17. Percentage of physicians in general practice and limited specialties by geographic divisions. In: Factual data on medical economics. Chicago, IL: American Medical Association; 1939.
18. Haug JN. Federal and nonfederal physicians in United States and possessions by specialty and activity, December 31, 1970. In: Haug JN, Roback GA, Martin BC. Distribution of physicians in the United States, 1970; regional, state, county, metropolitan areas. Chicago, IL: American Medical Association; 1971.
19. National Center for Health Statistics: physician visits, volume and interval since last visit, United States, 1971. DHEW Publication No. (HRA) 75-1524, Series 10, No. 97. US Printing Office, Washington, D.C., 1975; (a) Page 49.

20. Hoffman B. Emergency rooms: the reluctant safety net. In: Stevens RA, Rosenberg CE, Burns LR. Putting the past back in: history and health policy in the United States. New Brunswick, NJ: Rutgers University Press; 2006. p. 256.
21. Block LE. Evolution, growth and status of managed care in the United States. Pub Health Rev 1997; 25:193-244.
22. Silver MH. The emergency department problem. JAMA 1966;198:146-49.
23. Springall WH. The hospital emergency room. Ariz Med 1964; 21:661-2.
24. Committee on Medical Facilities, American Medical Association. Report on physician-hospital relations. Chicago: American Medical Association; 1964.
25. Davis J. How the US automobile industry has changed. Investopedia Academy. [cited 02 May 2017]. Available from: http://www.investopedia.com/articles/pf/12/auto-industry.asp
26. World Health Organisation. Road traffic injuries. [Fact Sheet]. Geneva; 2016 [cited 02 May 02 2017]. Available from: http://www.who.int/mediacentre/factsheets/fs358/en/
27. National Academy of Sciences/National Research Council: Accidental death and disability: the neglected disease of modern society. Washington, DC, 1966.
28. Pautz M. Decline in average weekly cinema attendance, 1930-2000. Issues in Political Economy. 2002;11.
29. McIntosh HD. The maturation of a cardiologist with reflections on the "Passing Sands of Time." Ann Emerg Med 1986;15:1101-10.
30. Montagu I: The political censorship of films. London: Victor Gollancz, Ltd; 1929.
31. Ibid. p 31.
32. Editorial. How authentic is medicine on television? JAMA 1957;164:49-51.
33. Turow J. Playing doctor: television, storeytelling, and medical power. Ann Arbor: University of Michigan Press; 2010. p. 59.
34. Dux S: The Citadel (1938): doctors, censors and the cinema. Hist J Film Radio Television 2012;32:1-17.
35. Immediate counterattack. Time. 1967 Sept1; 90(9):32.
36. Ludmerer K. Time to heal: American Medical Education from the turn of the century to the era of managed care. New York: Oxford University Press; 1999. p.335.
37. Hoffman B. Emergency rooms: the reluctant safety net. In: Stevens RA, Rosenberg CE, Burns LR. Putting the past back in: history and

health policy in the United States. New Brunswick, NJ: Rutgers University Press; 2006. p. 252.

38. Altman D, Frist WH. Medicare and Medicaid at 50 Years: perspectives of beneficiaries, health care professionals. JAMA 2015;314:384-95.

39. National Health Service. London. The history of the NHS in England. 2015 Jul 6 [cited 03 May 2017]; Available from: http://www.nhs.uk/NHSEngland/thenhs/nhshistory/Pages/NHShistory1948.aspx

40. Health Canada. Ottawa. Canada's health care system. 2012 Oct 09 [cited 03 May 2017]; Available from: http://www.hc-sc.gc.ca/hcs-sss/pubs/system-regime/2011-hcs-sss/index-eng.php

41. Curran WJ. Legal history of emergency medicine from medieval common law to the AIDS epidemic. Am J Emerg Med 1997;15:658-70.

42. Nahum LH. The emergency room. Conn Med 1965;29:760-63.

43. Rosen P. History of emergency medicine. In: Bowles LT, Sirica CM. The role of emergency medicine in the future of American medical care: A conference sponsored by the Josiah Macy, Jr. Foundation, Williamsburg, VA, April 17-20, 1994. New York: Josiah Macy, Jr. Foundation; 1995: p. 59-79.

44. American College of Surgeons. Hospital emergency facilities and services: A survey. Bull Am Coll Surg 1961; 46:44-50.

45. Larrey D-J. Mémoires de chirurgie militaire et campagnes. Paris: J Smith; 1812.

46. Manring MM, Hawk A, Calhoun JH, Andersen RC. Treatment of war wounds: a historical review. Clin Orthop Relat Res 2009 467: 2168–91.

47. Haacker LP, Time and its effects on casualties in World War II and Vietnam. Arch Surg 1969; 98:39-40.

48. Shah MN. The formation of the emergency medical services system. Am J Pub Health 2006; 96:414-23.

49. Howard JM. Historical background to Accidental Death and Disability: The Neglected Disease of Modern Society. Prehosp Emerg Care 2000;4:285-89.

50. National Academy of Sciences/National Research Council. Accidental death and disability: the neglected disease of modern society. Washington, DC; National Academy of Sciences, 1966.

Chapter 2

Development of cardio-pulmonary resuscitation, defibrillation and hospital coronary care units

Early attempts to organise resuscitation services originated with the need to revive people after submersion in water, at a time when many young healthy sailors were lost to drowning. This developed in the late 18th century with the formation of Humane Societies in Europe, Britain and the USA - starting in 1767 in Amsterdam with its extensive canal network.[1] These societies established registries to document the number of successful 'reanimations' and to promote effective resuscitation techniques. They advocated clearing the airway, mouth-to-mouth respiration and warming the victim; all good advice – only to lose some credibility with the directive to insufflate the rectum with tobacco smoke. The Dutch society even developed a fumigating apparatus for this purpose; it was thought that the 'nervous stimulation' induced by the tobacco would add restorative benefit.[1]

Mouth-to-mouth ventilation soon fell from favour: William Hunter dismissed it as *'a method practiced by the vulgar'* and Herholdt and Rafn considered *'insufflation of air by mouth is a very toilsome and loathsome act'*. [2,3] Apart from the aesthetic aspects, expired air was felt to be harmful due to its high carbon dioxide content. The bellows technique of ventilation, advocated by John Hunter,[4] was preferred until the mid 1800s when mechanical methods aimed at inducing respiratory movements of the chest wall were introduced – of which the Silvester and Holger Nielsen techniques had the widest acceptance.[5-7]

Airway and Breathing

It would take the sustained efforts of an American anaesthetist, James Elam, to restore mouth-to-mouth ventilation as the method of choice for resuscitation. In 1946, before his training in anaesthesia, Elam was responsible for the care of paralysed polio patients in Minneapolis. During temporary lapses in the function of tank respirators ('iron lung') he would sustain the patients with mouth-to-mouth or mouth-to-nose ventilation.[8]

Later as a research anaesthetist at Barnes Hospital in St Louis, Missouri, he carried out his definitive study demonstrating that mouth-to-mouth or mouth-to-tracheal tube ventilation could maintain normal arterial blood gas levels.[9] A chance meeting between Elam and Peter Safar, at that time the chief of anaesthesia at the Baltimore City Hospital, took place in October 1956 at the American Society of Anesthesiologists meeting in Kansas City – or more specifically following the meeting, during a shared car trip from Kansas to Chicago. Elam convinced Safar of the efficacy of expired air ventilation, which launched Safar on his ground-breaking research into methods of resuscitation and led to a life-long intellectual collaboration between the two men.[8,10]

The first piece of Safar's research was to find a practical way to overcome the airway obstruction from the tongue and soft tissues that occurs in the unconscious patient. Safar showed that this could be prevented in most cases by the simple head tilt and chin lift method – a technique he had seen used by anaesthetists in his early days in Austria.[10-12]

The next phase of his research was among the most audacious ever undertaken and would change both the method of ventilation for resuscitation and establish that modern resuscitation techniques could be effectively applied by laypersons. In 1957 Safar recruited local physicians and medical students to act as subjects to compare the efficacy of manual methods of ventilation to that of the mouth-to-mouth technique. To do this he sedated and then paralysed the subjects with succinyl choline. This he carried out on the floor of his hospital's operating theatre on Saturdays. Tidal volume and oximeter readings were compared for the various methods of ventilation. The manual methods were carried out by trained rescuers from the Baltimore City Fire Department and the mouth-to-mouth technique by lay volunteers, including boy scouts – all of whom received just one live demonstration on a subject by Safar himself. The results established the clear superiority of mouth-to-mouth ventilation and that this could easily be mastered by lay persons.[10, 13,14] Commenting later on the principle of informed consent and the lack of institutional review boards Safar wrote '.....I and other resuscitation researchers studied patients and human volunteers by assuming personal responsibility and seeking approval only from our local peers.'[10]

Circulation

Establishing an airway and ventilation could provide adequate resuscitation if the heart was still beating, but would be of no avail unless cardiac action circulated oxygenated blood to the vital organs – particularly the heart and brain. In the 19th century most witnessed cardiac arrests were caused by anaesthetic agents in operating theatres. The response to cardiac standstill could involve direct cardiac massage either through the diaphragm via an abdominal incision or directly via thoracotomy. Moritz Schiff of Florence, Italy was the first to demonstrate this in experiments on dogs in 1874.[15] Direct open-chest cardiac massage became the favoured response to cardiac arrest during the first half of the 20th century, with a success rate of about 25%.[15]

The evolution of closed-chest cardiac massage was more insidious, and once again the early application involved cases of cardiac arrest complicating chloroform anaesthesia. One of the earliest reports came from Janos Balassa, Professor of Surgery at the University of Pest in Hungary. In 1858 he published a case report of a young woman with obstructive laryngeal tuberculosis in whom he performed a tracheotomy. Her heart stopped and he wrote, *'I began to apply a rhythmic pressure to the chest simulating breathing;'* the patient recovered.[16] Although Balassa was merely trying to produce respiratory movements, there may well have been an element of cardiac compression associated with his efforts. In 1892 Friedrich Maass, surgical assistant to Professor Franz Koenig of Gottingen, reported two cases of successful sustained chest compressions in chloroform-related cardio-respiratory arrest.[17] Once again, Maass was attempting to apply respiratory assistance but his description was similar to that of modern chest compressions and he noted that his efforts produced carotid pulsations.[18,19] Experiments with chloroform-overdosed cats by Professor Boehm of Dorpat in 1878 showed that sternal compressions could sustain adequate blood pressure and carotid artery blood flow.[19] In 1904, George Crile, a surgeon in Cleveland, successfully resuscitated a woman who collapsed under anaesthesia. He used external chest compressions which he felt produced a *'pseudo-cardiac movement'* and which caused *'a pulse in the radial artery and bleeding of the peripheral vessels.'*[19]

As already noted, the first half of the 20th century was dominated by open chest cardiac massage and the few, isolated reports of closed chest compression were ignored or not recorded in sufficiently widespread publications.

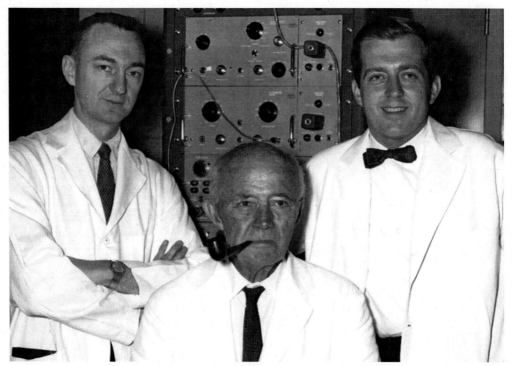

Fig 2.1 Left to right: James Jude (1928-2015) William Kouwenhoven (1886-1975) and Guy Knickerbocker (1932-)

Meanwhile at the Johns Hopkins University in Baltimore an unusual trio of two electrical engineers (William Kouwenhoven and Guy Knickerbocker) and a cardiac surgery resident (James Jude), were to conduct a series of studies that would help rediscover external cardiac massage and, ultimately, combine it with the airway and breathing techniques that made it possible to sustain cardiac arrest victims until defibrillation was available (see later).(Figure 2.1)

It would take the serendipitous observation by the prepared mind of Guy Knickerbocker to 'rediscover' the effectiveness of external, closed chest, cardiac massage. During their experiments to defibrillate dogs the paddles were modified, as a safety feature, to require fifteen pounds of pressure before the current would discharge. Knickerbocker observed that when the paddles were applied to the chest with the requisite force there was a spike in the dog's peripheral arterial pressure.[19, 20] Further observations led them to apply the pressure with their hands and they ultimately discovered that the best technique was rhythmic pressure on the lower sternum with the heel of the hand. By using repeated chest compressions in this manner they were able to extend the period of time that the dog could be sustained until successful defribrillation.[20,21] They published these results in 1960[21] and Jude later emulated and collated these results in the clinical arena.[22]

Thus, the **A**irway and **B**reathing aspects of resuscitation were established by 1958 and the **C**irculation component by 1960-61. It was to be the chief of the Baltimore Fire Department, Martin McMahon, who helped provide the spark that brought together the work of the two separate academic units in Baltimore.[19] Peter Safar had provided training for McMahon and his firemen and involved them in his studies of airway and breathing techniques.[10,19] Jude showed McMahon his chest compression data, who then insisted that his firemen learn both techniques. Safar was also quick to realise the necessity of all three components, the AB and C, in providing basic life support – or Cardiopulmonary Resuscitation (CPR) as it came to be known.[23] The final component of the ABCD resuscitation package was **D**efibrillation and the role of the **A**irway **B**reathing and **C**irculation was to sustain the victim until defibrillation was available.

Defibrillation

During the early decades of the twentieth century a growing incidence of sudden unexpected deaths occurring in the community had become a serious problem. High voltage shocks were a fairly common occurrence in the expanding electricity industry: electrical discharges of a strength greater than about forty volts were capable of precipitating fatal cardiac arrest by activating the muscle fibres in the ventricles, the heart's main pumping chambers, and causing them to contract in a completely haphazard, desynchronised and useless fashion ('ventricular fibrillation'), with no effective resulting heart beat.[24]

Another recognised cause of unexpected sudden deaths during the same era arose, during surgical operations, from an 'idiosyncratic' cardiac response to the use of certain anaesthetic agents, of which chloroform was the principal culprit. This 'idiosyncratic' response was ultimately found to be ventricular fibrillation.[25]

The other cause of cardiac arrest was the acute coronary attack. During ventricular fibrillation there is no pulse or audible heartbeat and therefore the cardiac 'arrest' was assumed to be due to asystole. In 1889, John McWilliam, Professor of Medicine at Aberdeen, established that in the majority of such cases it was ventricular fibrillation, or ventricular 'delirium' as he called it. '…..*the ventricles are thrown into a tumultuous state of quick, irregular, twitching action…..The ventricles become distended with blood, as the rapid quivering movement of their walls is wholly insufficient to expel their contents*'.[26-28]

In all of these causes of cardiovascular collapse: electrocution, anaesthesia-related and the acute coronary attack, the common denominator was ventricular fibrillation. Unless the fibrillation resolved spontaneously within a short time (a rare event), death was inevitable. The cardiac defibrillator (which would have the potential, by releasing a powerful shock through the ventricular muscle, to make the individual fibres contract synchronously 'in step' once again and restore the circulation of oxygenated blood) had not yet been developed. Unrecognised was the work of the Geneva physiologists Jean-Louis Prevost and Frederic Battelli in 1899. After inducing ventricular fibrillation in dogs by temporarily occluding the left coronary artery, they recorded the effects of both alternating (AC) and direct (DC) current on the arrhythmia. They found that both currents, when applied through the chest wall, could convert the ventricular fibrillation to sinus rhythm and DC was superior to AC.[29] However, neither they or their readership related these results to sudden death in humans, despite the work of McWilliam reported ten years earlier.

Development of defibrillators

During the third decade of the twentieth century some of the electrical supply companies in the United States sought advice on finding a solution to the alarming number of fatal accidents involving electric shocks which were occurring in their industry. The upshot was that the Rockefeller Institute funded research at a number of universities of which Johns Hopkins was one. Important work relevant to the problem was performed there by two physicians, Orthello Langworthy and Donald Hooker, and an electrical engineer, William Kouwenhoven. During the course of their research on anaesthetised dogs, they were able to show that even relatively minor shocks applied to the chest could initiate ventricular fibrillation, and that this could be corrected by stronger shocks applied after a short delay – 'countershock' as they called it.[30,31] Perhaps their most important (and encouraging) observation was that it was possible to terminate fibrillation and restore normal heart function in the dogs by means of a promptly applied external shock, without the need to open the chest.[30] It is probable that, on the basis of the results of these experiments, researchers were encouraged some fifteen years later to persist with attempts to prove that external defibrillation without thoracotomy would be practicable in humans.

The Second World War interrupted research into the development of defibrillators but, shortly before the war began, Claude Beck, Professor of Surgery at the Cleveland Western Reserve University, impressed by the tragic and seemingly unnecessary and wasteful loss of life caused by intra-operative ventricular fibrillation, himself built a defibrillator and subsequently achieved temporary successes with it on two patients who developed ventricular fibrillation during thoracic surgery.[32] Although the hearts of both patients functioned for only a short time after they were resuscitated, these events represented an important 'proof of principle': survival from this previously uniformly and immediately fatal disturbance of rhythm was undoubtedly possible. He was determined that, as he put it, hearts that were *'too good to die'* would, in the relatively near future, be able to survive.[33] In the *'nothing new under the sun'* category, it is of interest that some seventy years before Beck's classic and oft-quoted description of 'hearts too good to die' John McWilliam also had noted that in many of the sudden cardiac deaths there was no discernible pathology of the heart: *'But sudden stoppage of the heart's action has often been observed apart from the occurrence of gross structural lesions,.....not infrequently the cardiac substance has exhibited no pronounced morbid change.'* [27]

In 1947 Dr. Beck was able to achieve complete success with the defibrillation and subsequent long term survival of a fourteen year old boy upon whom he was operating for the correction of a disabling 'funnel chest' deformity.[34] Apart from an episode of sustained rapid heart action, the operation went well but, towards the end, the youth unexpectedly developed ventricular fibrillation which persisted for some forty-five minutes while Beck's bulky defibrillator was brought from another building. Dr. Beck, who had been providing internal cardiac massage, now delivered two shocks in sequence directly to the fibrillating heart through sterile metal 'paddles'. Fortunately an effective ventricular rhythm with an arterial pulse was restored by the second of these. The boy's condition became stable and he subsequently made a complete recovery.[34] This event represented not only the first record of the long term survival of a human resuscitated from ventricular fibrillation, but it also documented the possibility of transporting a defibrillator over some distance in order to provide its life-saving therapy, while appropriate 'first aid' ABC treatment sustained the patient.

During the 1950s more powerful, and unavoidably heavier, machines weighing of the order of 250-270 lb were constructed for external use on humans. William Kouwenhoven (who by now had experience of defibrillation - albeit interrupted by the war - over a period spanning twenty years), and Paul Zoll of Boston (who had in 1952 developed the first external cardiac pacemaker for use on patients who had an abnormally slow - or at times temporarily absent - heartbeat), were both interested

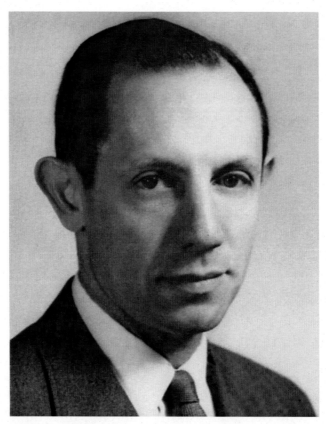

Fig 2.2 Paul Zoll (1911-1999). The Boston cardiologist was the first to show that the heart could be defibrillated by a shock across the closed chest.

in developing defibrillators capable of correcting ventricular fibrillation through the intact human chest wall.[35] (Figure 2.2) Each of the machines they designed would deliver high voltage alternating current shocks (of the order of 480 to 1000 volts for adults). One metal 'paddle' smeared with conductive gel would be pressed firmly against the front surface of the right upper chest and the other, similarly treated with gel, would be held in contact with the skin over the 'cardiac apex' on the left side, centred on the space just below the fifth rib. An electric shock administered with the paddles in these positions would ensure that the highest possible density of the resulting current would be concentrated within the main muscle mass of the heart.

Dr. Zoll's ungainly defibrillator was ready for use in the second half of 1955 and it was used in the attempted resuscitation of four patients between late August and mid-November. It successfully removed ventricular fibrillation in all four. Only the fourth patient survived, but this technical success represented the needed 'proof of principle'.[36,37] Dr. Kouwenhoven's similarly heavy defibrillator was first used on human patients in 1957: the first patient to be treated required defibrillation on multiple occasions and did not survive to leave hospital. The second patient developed ventricular fibrillation during a diagnostic test -probably cardiac catheterisation. Defibrillation was performed just over one minute later and was immediately successful in restoring a stable circulation leading to her long-term survival.[38]

These large defibrillators (which employed alternating current for defibrillation and required a heavy transformer to reach the required voltage), had the obvious drawback of limited portability. Dr. Kouwenhoven had at one time considered the possibility of employing DC defibrillation using a charge stored on a capacitor, but initial animal experiments performed with it had yielded unsatisfactory results. This finding did not necessarily rule out the possibility that the configuration (or waveform) of a direct current shock might be modulated, or 'shaped', in such a way as to make it capable of terminating fibrillation. An unmodified high voltage direct current discharge emanating from a capacitor through a conducting medium having a relatively low electrical resistance (such as the human torso) will naturally be very short in duration (because of rapid depletion of the charge on the capacitor), in contrast to that of a single half cycle emanating from an alternating current source which, at the standard frequency (in the United States) of sixty cycles per second, would have a duration of 8.5 milliseconds. (In the United Kingdom, where the standard frequency is fifty cycles per second, the corresponding half cycle duration would be 10 milliseconds). A 'pure' direct current capacitor discharge (without an essential inductor coil being included in the circuit) would have a much shorter duration, in the region of 1-2 milliseconds, too brief to result in defibrillation.

As a result of their size and weight these machines were really only suitable for situations in which the patients for whom they might be required could be grouped together within a relatively small area (and ideally connected to some form of electrocardiographic monitoring) making it possible for the hospital staff to perform defibrillation promptly if required, without the need to move the defibrillator more than a few metres. For those patients who were fortunate enough to develop ventricular fibrillation within easy reach of a defibrillator, this scenario offered the prospect of prompt correction of the fibrillation delivered through the intact chest wall. This arrangement could be considered to represent the 'lowest common denominator' for what was destined to develop into the 'Coronary Care Unit'.

In order to cover situations in which a defibrillator was not immediately available, some physicians and surgeons made a point, during the late 1950s, of carrying a scalpel and sterile gloves around with them so that they could open the chest and provide direct cardiac massage promptly should they encounter a patient immediately after the onset of cardiac arrest. A cardiologist from the United Kingdom, Desmond Julian, who was working in Australia at the time, and who was soon to become a prominent figure in the field of acute coronary care, was among those who for a time adopted this approach. Julian also recounted the incident of the Dean of Medicine at Johns Hopkins recovering from a faint, only to find a colleague poised over him with a scalpel at the ready.[39]

Evolution of the Resuscitation Protocol

As is often the case in medicine, progress tends to be influenced substantially by immediate practicalities relating to what is available, rather than by theoretically ideal solutions. The Johns Hopkins trio of two engineers, Kouwenhoven and Knickerbocker, and a surgical trainee, Jude, performed their studies on the closed-chest induction and termination of ventricular fibrillation in anaesthetised dogs in a laboratory which was situated in the same building in which Dr. Jude at other times undertook his surgical duties. With regard to the research on anaesthetised dogs, they developed a good grasp of the interval for which they could safely leave the animals in a state of cardiac arrest before a defibrillatory 'rescue' shock became mandatory for their survival. Probably as a result of the co-existence of resuscitation research and clinical surgical activities in the same institution, these individuals were able to make dramatic progress in the field of resuscitation medicine within a remarkably short period of time.

The widespread dissemination of the technique of mouth-to-mouth artificial respiration, along with external cardiac massage, resulted in a dramatic increase in the number of patients 'rescued' from cardiac arrest. The technique of CPR was crystalised at conferences on Cardiopulmonary Resuscitation held in the United States in 1966 and in Norway in 1967. In order to facilitate the teaching of CPR, as early as 1958, a Norwegian doll maker, Asmund Laerdal, was approached by Peter Safar with a view to producing a training mannequin for CPR to facilitate widespread dissemination of the resuscitation technique.(Figure 2.3) The result was the universally known 'Resusci-Anne' mannequin.[40] (Figure 2.4)

28

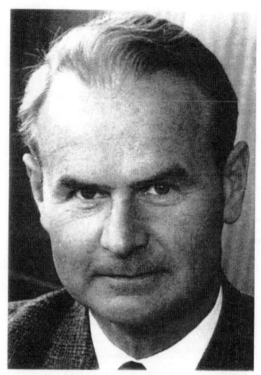

Fig 2.3 Asmund Laerdal (1913-1981)

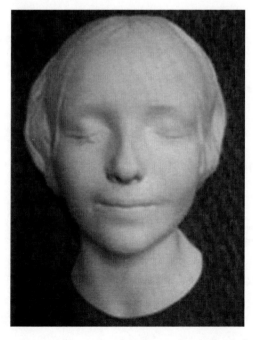

Fig 2.4 Resusci Anne. Based on the death mask of a girl drowned in the River Seine, Paris

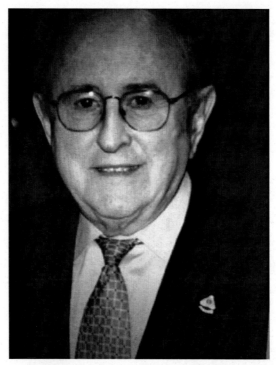

Fig 2.5 Bernard Lown (1921-   )

A Better Defibrillator

In 1962, Bernard Lown, a cardiologist in Boston, gained access to a defibrillator which gave direct current (DC) shocks.[41,42] (Figure 2.5) Access to this machine arose because of an agreement between the United States and Russia to share medically significant information which could be of universal value in treating disease. The circuitry had been created and tested in animals by Dr. Naum Gurvich in Moscow some twenty years earlier.[43,44] Briefly, the unacceptably short duration of a simple capacitor discharge had been prolonged in a controlled fashion by placing a condenser in the circuit (the precise waveform depending on the properties of the condenser). An additional feature of this machine was that it was now possible to synchronise the shock with the electrocardiogram in such a way that it would only release a shock in conjunction with a detected 'R' wave on the electrocardiogram, a feature which meant that the defibrillator could also be used to treat non-lethal arrhythmias such as atrial fibrillation and ventricular tachycardia. In a study comparing alternating and direct defibrillators Lown found that DC was safer and more effective at correcting arrhythmias than AC.[42]

Although the circuitry of the initial direct current defibrillator resulted in a weight only modestly less than that of existing AC defibrillators, there was the potential to produce a modified device specifically for treating cardiac arrest without incorporating a synchroniser. More importantly, the subsequent development of lighter charging circuitry and smaller capacitors would make it possible to reduce the weight considerably, leading to more portable defibrillators and, eventually, a machine which could be implanted inside the human body.

Coronary Care Units

Surgeons were the first to create and realise the benefits of concentrating technical and human resources to improve outcome in sick postoperative patients. This was of special relevance to postoperative cardiac surgery in the 1940-50s. As technical supports for critically ill patients became available (respirators, cardiac monitors, artificial kidney machines) the development of special care units, along with specially trained medical and nursing staff, yielded improved outcomes.[45] The ability to diagnose, monitor and treat arrhythmias (including the fatal ventricular fibrillation) associated with myocardial infarction led to the establishment of special 'coronary care units.' These units concentrated the resources of cardiac monitors, defibrillator and constant nursing staff trained in CPR and defibrillation – backed by suitably trained medical staff.[45]

The first two such coronary care units (CCU) were set up in Edinburgh by Desmond Julian, at that time a senior cardiology resident, and in Kansas City, Kansas by cardiologist Hughes Day; reported in 1961 and 1962 respectively.[46,47] It is salutary to find that these first two reports on CCUs did not gain easy access to publication; Julian was first rejected by the *British Medical Journal* and Day published in the obscure *Journal-Lancet* because none of the mainstream journals were interested in his manuscript.[45,48] CCUs were set up in Philadelphia and Toronto at about the same time and, as the 1960s progressed, soon became established in most major hospitals.[49]

The value of these units became apparent as the hospital mortality after acute myocardial infarction fell from 30% with general hospital care to less than 20% with intensive care in CCUs.[50,51] The majority of this mortality reduction was due to the detection and successful treatment of potentially fatal cardiac arrhythmias, including ventricular fibrillation.[50]

References

1. Sternbach GL, Varon J, Fromm R, Baskett PJF. The Humane Societies. Resuscitation 2000;45:71-5.
2. Hernholdt JD, Rafn CG. An Attempt at an Historical Survey of Life-saving Measures for Drowning Persons. Copenhagen: H. Tikiob & M. Seest; 1796.
3. Baskett PJF. JD Hernholdt and CG Rafn: two unsung heroes from Denmark. Resuscitation 2007;74:8-10.
4. Hunter J. Proposal for the recovery of people apparently drowned. Phil Trans R Soc London 1776.
5. Silvester HR. A new method of resuscitating still-born children, and of restoring the persons apparently drowned or dead. BMJ 1858;2:576-9.
6. Baskett TF. Silvester's technique of artificial respiration. Resuscitation 2007;74:8-10.
7. Baskett TF. The Holger Nielsen method of artificial respiration. Resuscitation 2007;74:403-5.
8. Safar P. James O. Elam. Resuscitation 2001;50:249-56.
9. Elam JO, Brown ES, Elder JD. Artificial respiration by mouth-to-mask method. A study of the respiratory gas exchange of paralyzed patients ventilated by the operators exhaled air. N Engl J Med 1954;250:749-54.
10. Baskett PJF. Peter Safar, the early years 1924-1961, the birth of CPR. Resuscitation 2001;50:17-22.
11. Safar P. Mouth to mouth airway. Anesthesiology 1957;18:904-6.
12. Safar P. Ventilatory efficacy of mouth-to-mouth artificial respiration. Airway obstruction during manual and mouth-to-mouth artificial respiration. JAMA 1958;167:335-41.
13. Safar P, Escarraga L, Elam J. A comparison of the mouth-to-mouth and mouth-to-airway methods of artificial respiration with the chest-pressure arm-lift methods N Engl J Med 1958;258:671-7.
14. Safar P, Elam J. Manual versus mouth-to-mouth methods of artificial respiration. Anesthesiology 1958;19:111-2.
15. Vallejo-Manzur F, Varon J, Fromm R, Baskett P. Moritz Schiff and the history of open-chest cardiac massage. Resuscitation 2002;53:3-5.
16. Baskett TF, Kis M. Janos Balassa and resuscitation by chest compression. Resuscitation 2005;65:11-13.
17. Maass F. Die method der wiederbelebung bei herztod nach chloroformeinathmung. Berlin Klin Wochenschr 1982;12:265-8.
18. Figl M, Pelinka LE, Mauritz W. Franz Koenig and Friedrich Maass.

Resuscitation 2006;70:6-9.

19. Eisenberg M. Life in the Balance. New York: Oxford University Press;1997.p109-129.

20. Acosta P, Varon J, Sternbach GL, Baskett P. Kouwenhoven, Jude and Knickerbocker: the introduction of defibrillation and external chest compressions into modern resuscitation. Resuscitation 2005;64:139-43.

21. Kouwenhoven WB, Jude J, Knickerbocker G. Closed chest cardiac massage. JAMA 1960;173:1064-7.

22. Jude J, Kouwenhoven WB, Knickerbocker G. Cardiac arrest; report of application of external cardiac massage on 118 patients. JAMA 1961;178:1063-71.

23. Safar P, Brown TC, Holtey WH. Ventilation and circulation with closed chest cardiac massage in man. JAMA 1961;176:574-6.

24. Cunningham RH. The cause of death from industrial electric currents. NY Med J 1899;69:622.

25. Levy AG, Lewis T. Heart irregularities resulting from the inhalation of low percentages of chloroform vapour, and their relationship to ventricular fibrillation. Heart 1911;3:99.

26. McWilliam JA. Fibrillar contraction of the heart. J Physiol 1887;8:296-310.

27. McWilliam JA. Cardiac failure and sudden death. BMJ 1889;1:6-8.

28. Filho FE, Chamberlain D. John Alexander McWilliam. Resuscitation 2006;69:3-7.

29. Prevost JL, Battelli F. La mort par le courant électrique – courant alternatifs a haute tension. J Physiol Path Gen 1899;1:427-42.

30. Hooker DR, Kouwenhoven WB, Langworthy OR. The effect of alternating electrical currents on the heart. Am J Physiol 1933;103:444-54.

31. Kouwenhoven WB, Hooker DR. Resuscitation by countershock. Electrical Engineering 1933:475-7.

32. Beck CS. Resuscitation for cardiac standstill and ventricular fibrillation occurring during operation. Am J Surg 1941;54:273-9.

33. Beck CS, Leighniger DS. Death after a clean bill of health. JAMA 1960;174:133-5.

34. Beck CS, Pritchard WH, Feil HS. Ventricular fibrillation of long duration abolished by electric shock. JAMA 1947;135:985-6.

35. Zoll P. Resuscitation of the heart in ventricular standstill by external electrical stimulation. N Engl J Med 1952;247:761-71.

36. Zoll P, Linenthal AJ, Norman LR, Paul MH, Gibson W. Treatment of unexpected cardiac arrest by external electric stimulation of the

heart. N Engl J Med 1956;254:541-6.

37. Zoll PM, Linenthal AJ, Gibson W, Paul MH, Norman LR . Termination of ventricular fibrillation in man by externally applied countershock. N Engl J Med 1956;254:727-32.

38. Kouwenhoven WB, Milnor WR, Knickerbocker GG et al. Closed chest defibrillation of the heart. Surgery 1957;42:550-61.

39. Julian DG. The evolution of the coronary care unit. Cardiovascular Research. 2001;51:621-4.

40. Tjomsland N, Baskett P. Asmund S. Laerdal. Resuscitation 2002;53:115-9.

41. Eisenberg M. Bernard Lown and defibrillation. Resuscitation 2006;69:171-3.

42. Lown B, Neuman J, Amarasingham R, Berkovits BV. Comparison of alternating current with direct current electroshock across the closed chest. Am J Cardiol 1962;223-33.

43. Gurvich NL, Yunier G. Restoration of regular rhythm in the mammalian fibrillating heart. Bull Exp Biol Med 1939;8:55-8. (In Russian) English translation in Am Rev Sov Med 1946;3:236-9.

44. Ussenko LV, Tsarev AV, Leschenko YA. Naum L Gurvich: a pioneer of defibrillation. Resuscitation 2006;70:170-2.

45. Fye WB. American Cardiology: The History of a Specialty and its College. Baltimore: Johns Hopkins University Press;1996.p176-81.

46. Julian DG. Treatment of cardiac arrest in acute myocardial ischaemia and infarction. Lancet 1961;2:840-4.

47. Day HW. A cardiac resuscitation program. Journal-Lancet 1962;82:153-6.

48. Silverman ME. Desmond Gareth Julian: Pioneer in Coronary Care. In: Profiles in Cardiology. Hurst JW, Conti CR, Fye WB(eds). Mahwah, NJ: Foundation for Advances in Medicine and Science; 2003.p474-5.

49. Day HW. History of coronary care units. Am J Cardiol 1972;30:405-7.

50. Lown B, Fakhro AM, Hood WB, Thorn GW. The coronary care unit: new perspectives and directions. JAMA 1967;199:188-93.

51. Lawrie DM, Greenwood TW, Harvey AC et al. A coronary care unit in the routine management of acute myocardial infarction. Lancet 1967;2:109-11.

Chapter 3

Belfast gets the message

John Stafford Geddes qualified in Medicine in June 1963 and on 1st August he started his first three month rotation as a House Physician ('Houseman') with an attachment to Dr. Frank Pantridge, Senior Consultant Physician in Wards 5 and 6 on the main corridor of the Royal Victoria Hospital, Belfast (RVH). (Figure 3.1)

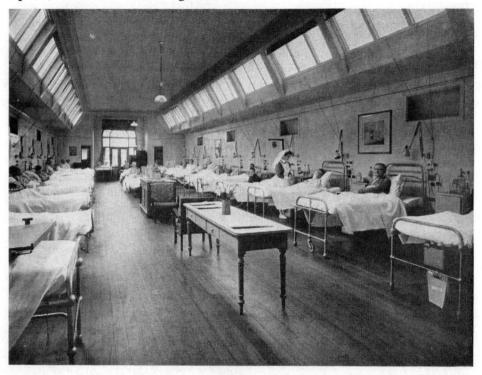

Fig 3.1
Ward 6, Royal Victoria Hospital, 1953.
In the late 1950s curtain rails were installed around each bed.

As a final year student Geddes had attended most of Dr. Pantridge's teaching rounds and therefore had a good idea of the variety of patients he was likely to see and the potential offered by recent medical advances for protecting them from complications which formerly might have proved fatal.

During his clinical attachments to other wards as a student he had encountered a number of patients admitted with acute heart attacks complicated either by reduced blood pressure associated with cold perspiration affecting the hands and feet (signs of 'cardiogenic shock'), or by shortness of breath accompanied by widespread tell-tale 'crackles' audible with a stethoscope held over their lungs (signifying 'heart failure', or a 'back-up' of fluid). Unfortunately, many of the patients exhibiting these signs did not respond to conventional treatment, and died within twenty-four to forty-eight hours. As a last ditch effort the doctor in charge would, not infrequently, administer an injection of a stimulant drug such as adrenaline or nikethamide directly into the heart through a fine needle - a treatment which could be nothing more than symbolic at that stage. Although occasional sudden and unexpected patient deaths did occur in the wards, in the absence of electrocardiographic monitoring it was uncommon for the initial collapse to be noticed. Often, in such cases, the bed screens were at least partially pulled across, making detection difficult. No defibrillator was available for use in the hospital wards and in general no attempt at resuscitation was made. Defibrillators, at least for internal use, were, however, available in the operating theatres for patients having thoracic procedures, including closed mitral valvotomy, and for paediatric cardiac surgery.

In September 1963, Dr. Pantridge attended a lecture in London given by Dr. Bernard Lown, a well-known American Cardiologist.[1] The lecture was on his experience with the direct current (DC) defibrillator which Lown had been using in Boston during the preceding two years. On his return to Belfast, Dr. Pantridge extolled the virtues of this machine during a morning coffee break. He emphasised an important safety feature in that it was fitted with a synchroniser which would prevent the administered shock from coinciding with the 'vulnerable period' during the T wave of the electrocardiogram, when provocation of ventricular fibrillation was likely.[2] This feature meant that it could be employed for elective conversion of non-lethal arrhythmias such as atrial fibrillation and stable ventricular tachycardia. Even as a junior doctor Geddes appreciated that Dr. Pantridge saw the defibrillator as having a dual role:

1. safe conversion of atrial fibrillation post mitral valvotomy, and
2. removing ventricular fibrillation in patients developing cardiac arrest.

The registrars (senior residents), were clearly most impressed with its potential uses.

Arrival of the defibrillator

Geddes' duties as house physician in Wards 5 and 6 came to an end on Thursday, 31st October, 1963. Just over a week earlier on Tuesday, 22nd October the 'Lown' defibrillator, of which Dr. Pantridge had spoken about a month previously, arrived amid much excitement among the staff. The company representative who accompanied it set up the large machine on a wheeled trolley, in a small side room off the entrance to Ward 6. (Figure 3.2).

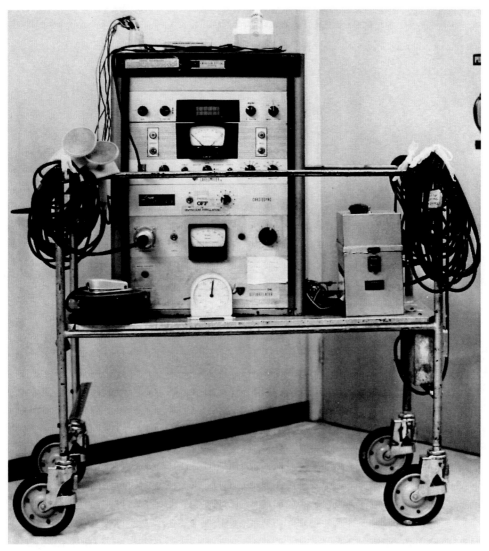

Fig 3.2
The Lown defibrillator arrived in Wards 5 and 6, RVH in October 1963

Dr. Pantridge, some of the registrars, Geddes, and Ward Sister Crawford were present. There was a relatively small screen high on the front of the defibrillator for monitoring the ECG and a larger screen below indicated the individual energy settings to be used. Lubricated metal paddles on the end of relatively long leads, held in contact with the front of the right upper chest and with the left side near the cardiac apex would be used to administer the shock. The representative described the functions of the various controls and in the course of conversation he mentioned that some of the doctors who had used the defibrillator to remove atrial fibrillation in the United States had found that quite small shocks were often adequate and, in fact, this treatment was often given with minimal or no sedation.

On the afternoon of Thursday, 24th October, 1963, Dr. Pantridge performed the hospital's first elective transthoracic electrical 'cardioversion.' The patient was a middle-aged woman who had persistent atrial fibrillation following a closed mitral valvotomy operation. In keeping with what he had been told by the company representative, Pantridge gave her a modest dose of diazepam ('valium') intravenously before he administered a moderate synchronised shock. The patient's heart rhythm was corrected and she was discharged about two hours later in good condition. She did, however have some choice words to say about the sensation she experienced with the new treatment – clearly the dose of diazepam was too small! This was the first elective 'Cardioversion' to be performed in Northern Ireland.

On Monday 28th October, 1963, Dr. Pantridge presented the details of the 'Lown' defibrillator and its significance at the weekly Physicians' Meeting held in the Old Surgical Extern (off the main RVH corridor). Dr. Pantridge outlined the new method of correcting cardiac arrhythmias by means of electrical discharges through the intact chest. He indicated that the new defibrillator, unlike the AC (alternating current) machines in use during the late 1950s, delivered a single, discreet, discharge through the patient's chest. The initial charge was stored on a capacitor and the discharge was released through an inductor coil designed in such a way that the duration of the shock was of the order of 5 milliseconds, and there was a smaller terminal portion of opposite polarity (the technical term was an 'underdamped biphasic discharge'). The peak voltage of the stored charge was some 2000 volts. A shock from this device had been shown to have a high probability of correcting ventricular fibrillation. Furthermore, unlike the previously available defibrillators which gave alternating current discharges, the exact timing of the shock could be set so as to avoid the 'vulnerable period' of the heart (a roughly 30 millisecond time window occurring within the 'T' wave during which a shock may cause ventricular fibrillation), when used for the correction of other, non-lethal, arrhythmias such as atrial fibrillation or ventricular tachycardia.[2]

Introduction of closed chest CPR at RVH

John Geddes first heard of this technique at about the time he qualified in Medicine in June, 1963, but does not recall receiving any formal instruction on closed chest resuscitation during the time he was a house physician in Wards 5 and 6. His next allocation in the hospital was the Casualty Department (ER), where he had a number of opportunities to witness attempted resuscitations and to become familiar with the technique. Three months later, when he arrived in the Neurosurgical Unit (NSU) in February, 1964, he had experience of observing and managing critically ill patients, including some who were in a state of cardiac arrest. These patients were placed in the supine position on a firm surface with one rescuer pressing firmly with the heels of both hands on the lower part of the sternum sufficiently hard to move it backwards two to three inches towards the spine at a rate of about sixty per minute. The lungs would be inflated by another rescuer once for every two to three chest compressions. This relatively low rate of chest compressions, recommended in the 1960s, was selected because of the erroneous belief that the venous pressure falls during cardiac arrest and that this lower pressure impedes cardiac filling during diastole – the time between successive compressions. By contrast, modern CPR specifies compressions at 120/min with 'rescue breaths' at two for every thirty compressions.

Start of the Royal Victoria Hospital Coronary Care Unit

Dr Pantridge began to speak of his intentions to open a Coronary Care Unit at least as early as August, 1963. He envisaged four beds with the patients in them all connected to a single oscilloscope through pads attached to their chests, which would be kept under constant observation 'by a roster of registrars and fellows'. There was little enthusiasm for this idea among the staff. Geddes, still involved in his internship in Neurosurgery, found time to visit the Cardiology wards, where on the evening of Monday 23rd December 1963 he was told that the prototype monitoring equipment had been installed during the previous week. The displays were on relatively small 'television' screens, one beside each bed. A nurse was sitting, keeping an eye on the tracings. No paper recording facilities were available. It was a start.

The CCU was 'unisex' situated on the male Ward 6. The four-bedded unit was later expanded to six and then eight beds.

Resuscitation after cardiac arrest performed outside the Neurosurgical Unit

One morning in late April, 1964, at about 11.00am Geddes was sitting in the Neurosurgical Clinical Room in Ward 21, RVH, having coffee with the consultants, registrars and Brian Pitt (the other house surgeon), when a hospital maintenance employee timidly opened the door and said, *'Excuse me, there is a man lying on the ground outside the building.'* Pitt and Geddes ran to the place where a middle-aged man had collapsed and on the way we called for help from other staff members. The victim was unresponsive. Geddes rolled him on his back, found that he had no pulse and started external cardiac massage. Several seconds later Dr Dennis Coppel, who was one of the two anaesthetists at that time working in the Neurosurgical Operating theatre, had emerged and was running towards the scene pushing an anaesthetic trolley. At his suggestion, Geddes paused the cardiac massage, permitting Coppel to intubate the victim and connect an oxygen supply. Cardiac massage was continued but the man remained pulseless and unconscious, although his colour had improved. It was decided to move the patient into the building, where we could obtain an electrocardiogram and further help. With the help of Anand Garg, Neurosurgical Registrar, we lifted the patient onto a trolley and, with CPR continuing, we wheeled him into the building and into a side ward. An ECG technician arrived and recorded the electrocardiogram, which showed ventricular fibrillation. It was notable that the amplitude of the fibrillation was quite large, indicative of the muscle of the patient's heart still being in relatively good condition. Geddes left the others to continue CPR while he went to telephone the cardiology ward.

Fortunately, Dr Pantridge was in Ward 6 and Geddes told him about the ongoing resusciatation attempt. Dr Pantridge agreed to come and see the patient, bringing with him the Lown defibrillator, accompanied by Dr Peter Halmos, a Research Fellow who was involved in a study of electrical cardioversion of atrial fibrillation among patients who had undergone mitral valvotomy surgery.

When they arrived, the defibrillator was plugged into the electrical socket and connected to the patient. The display screen confirmed continuing ventricular fibrillation. The electrolyte gel was spread over the paddles and, after ensuring that no-one was in contact with the patient, a shock (probably 400 Joules) was given. Fibrillation continued, but a second shock about 30 seconds later resulted in an organised rhythm with a palpable femoral pulse. A full electrocardiogram (ECG) was recorded and this now showed a supraventricular (probably sinus) rhythm with conspicuous elevation of the ST segment in the anterior leads. The patient's blood pressure was now recordable, with a systolic level of about 90mm. His respirations were adequate.

The patient was transferred to a bed in Ward 6 and connected to an ECG monitor. The 12 lead electrocardiogram there showed anterior ST segment elevation with loss of R waves consistent with a recent anterior myocardial infarction. Geddes returned to his duties in the Neurosurgical Unit but later that day visited the patient in Ward 6. He was in congestive heart failure but was reasonably comfortable while propped up in bed. His speech was incoherent and sadly he died during the night. It transpired that when he collapsed, he was on his way to an appointment at a medical outpatient clinic. This was the first documented case of successful, albeit temporary, resuscitation of a patient from ventricular fibrillation at the Royal Victoria Hospital.

Hospital cardiac arrest on call system

Geddes completed his intern rotations at the Royal Victoria Hospital on 31st July 1964, without any further direct involvement in cardio-pulmonary resuscitation. He returned the following day to Wards 5 and 6 as a Senior House Officer (junior resident) on 1st August. No detailed records relating to resuscitation attempts made since the episode occurring outside the Neurosurgery wards in April of that year were available, although the nursing staff indicated that a number of unsuccessful attempts had been made during this period.

Dr. Pantridge was determined that an effective mobile system should be developed for the immediate management of cardiac arrests occurring in any part of the hospital. The flat lay-out of Wards 1-20 (the majority of the medical and surgical units) along the main hospital corridor, with the Casualty (Accident and Emergency) Department also accessible on the same level, and with the Gynaecological and Neurosurgical/Neurological wards only a short distance further away than the main surgical units, meant that arranging 'universal' emergency access was much less challenging than would have been the case in the majority of hospitals, the architecture of which was based on the multi-storey principle. Only one three-storey building, comprising the Metabolic and Dermatology wards, exceeded two levels and this unit was easily accessible from a short zig-zag extension of the main hospital corridor beyond Ward 1. A further consideration was that it might become necessary to deal with two emergencies in different wards at the same time, and such an exigency would require a degree of redundancy and duplication of equipment.

The job of teaching the incoming junior medical staff the principles and techniques of CPR and defibrillation fell to Geddes and this is recounted by one such junior, Tom Baskett. In August 1964 Baskett started his houseman's (intern) year at the RVH. As a student 'living in' on the wards in the preceeding two years his only recollection of 'CPR' was the occasional, and always unsuccessful, attempt at intracardiac nikethamide injection. He witnessed and assisted at one thoracotomy and direct cardiac massage, carried out on the surgical ward; the patient was a postoperative man who arrested while Baskett and the senior resident were at his bedside. The attempted resuscitation failed and subsequent autopsy showed a massive pulmonary embolus.

Sometime that August, John Geddes, now the Senior House Officer on Wards 5 and 6, took each houseman (usually 1-3 at a time) for an introductory teaching session on the resuscitation cart and defibrillator in the side ward of Ward 6. He informed us that patients who had previously been said to have suddenly died would now be deemed to have 'cardiac arrest' and, in selected cases, could be resuscitated, defibrillated and saved. He outlined and demonstrated the components of modern CPR and how to work the defibrillator. There were no educational objectives or mission statements or, indeed, any written material. Merely a clear and practical guide on how to do it – lasting about 30 minutes. The additional skills of cut-down intravenous access (in those days not all patients in acute care beds had an IV in place) and endotracheal intubation, we had already acquired as students. Thereafter, we just got on with it and became quite proficient. As we lived in the hospital all the time (our official title was descriptively apt, Resident Medical Officer) we were inevitably the 'first responders' for all cases of cardiac arrest. Individual cases can have a lasting impact and one such served to confirm for me the value of this new approach to sudden death. A patient in his fifties, who I knew as the father of non-medical friends, was admitted with a myocardial infarction. The following day he arrested when we were close by, and therefore able to provide successful resuscitation. He went home and lived for many happy and productive years thereafter; this was the only case in which I had a personal link to provide long-term follow up.

The senior consulting medical staff (apart from Dr Pantridge) were not involved. Towards the end of the year Baskett was houseman to the Professor of Medicine, Graham Bull, on Wards 3 and 4. During the morning ward round a sixty year old woman, who had been admitted the night before on emergency 'take in' with a myocardial infarction, arrested in the bed next to us. The nurse and I went into our familiar and by now well-practiced routine; applied CPR and soon had her intubated and defibrillated. Professor Bull observed the whole scene with some bewilderment and, after we had the patient stabilised, he took me aside. 'Well done Baskett,' he said, 'that was impressive, but should I ever have a heart attack and cardiac arrest in your presence you must promise me that under no circumstances will you subject me to resuscitation.' He was deadly serious. The patient was discharged home two weeks later.[3]

The in-hospital resuscitation team consisted of one 'cardiac' Registrar and one House Physician who were available 'on call' in the hospital and carried pagers at all times. When necessary a more senior member of staff could be contacted. A Staff Nurse (RN) on duty in Wards 5 and 6 was also designated to respond to emergencies.

The main emergency cart carried the Cardioverter/Defibrillator, an Electrocardiograph machine with oscilloscope, a 'Stop Clock', and a supply of single-use needle electrodes in a jar of surgical spirit ready for use (at the time these needles were found to be the only reliable means of obtaining a clear electrocardiographic signal under 'cardiac arrest' conditions). A second cart, smaller in size, held a venous cut-down set and a torch (flash light) to provide adequate illumination at night. The equipment also included an Ambu Bag and mask, and intravenous solutions - 0.9% saline, 5% dextrose and 8.4% sodium bicarbonate – the latter considered essential to mitigate the adverse effect of metabolic acidosis on cardiac function. This cart also carried a laryngoscope, endotracheal tubes, an IV drip stand, and connecting rubber tubing for use with the other respiratory equipment. An assortment of needles with plastic sleeves for venous cannulation, instruments for venous cut-down with suitable cannulas, and a lumbar puncture needle for direct intracardiac injection of drugs (such as noradrenaline) were also available. Each morning Geddes arranged with the nursing staff that an intravenous set on this cart was run through with sodium bicarbonate, capped, and immediately available if required for a cardiac arrest occurring during the next twenty-four hours.

Towards the end of 1964 a second DC defibrillator was purchased and added to the second cart. This machine was similar in design and circuitry to the original defibrillator, except that it did not have an oscilloscopic display or a synchroniser which would allow it to be used for performing elective DC Cardioversions. However, it could deliver a direct current shock of up to 400 Joules, so it had the same potential for removing ventricular fibrillation as its 'fellow' machine. Thus, in the event of its being needed to treat a second patient in a state of cardiac arrest whilst the original machine

43

was in use elsewhere, it could be employed in conjunction with a separate oscilloscopic monitor (its circuitry protected from the shock by momentary disconnection from the patient) to remove ventricular fibrillation. For completeness, an external pacemaker for use with a transvenous catheter electrode was also carried on the second resuscitation trolley. With a maximum output of only about 10 volts it would have had to be used in conjunction with a transvenous electrode, either inserted previously and slightly displaced or 'blindly' inserted at the bedside. There was however no record of this being used in an emergency situation.

Outcome of cardiac arrest in hospital

By August 1964 the RVH in-hospital resuscitation programme was organised. The experience of the first eighteen months, up to February 1966, was reported in the Lancet later that year by Pantridge and Geddes.[4] (Figure 3.3)

At that time the published success rate of resuscitation after cardiac arrest in general medical wards was consistently poor – between 5 and 10%.[5-7] Over the 18 months studied, there were 50 cases of cardiac arrest in the RVH in whom the cardiac rhythm was recorded: 48 ventricular fibrillation and 2 asystole. Of these, 8 occurred in the CCU with a 62.5% long-term survival rate (discharge from hospital), whereas in the general wards the survival was 31%. However, even the latter figure was much better than the published survival rates, and they therefore concluded:

'The object of this report is to indicate that with adequate nursing instruction and a highly mobile resuscitation team, the chance of successful treatment, outside an intensive care unit, of cardiac arrest in patients with ischaemic heart disease, should be reasonably good.' [4]

They also noted, as a harbinger of future developments:

'Since the majority of deaths from cardiac arrest happen immediately after the onset of infarction, a mobile resuscitation team should be able to reach the patient in his own home.' (see chapter 4)

CARDIAC ARREST
AFTER MYOCARDIAL INFARCTION

J. F. PANTRIDGE
M.C., M.D. Belf., F.R.C.P.
PHYSICIAN

J. S. GEDDES
B.Sc., M.B. Belf.
SENIOR HOUSE-OFFICER

ROYAL VICTORIA HOSPITAL, BELFAST, 12

MORTALITY from cardiac arrest after myocardial infarction may be substantially reduced if patients are admitted to intensive-care units. Julian et al. (1964) and Day (1965) reported successful resuscitation in 40% and 54%, respectively, of patients who had a cardiac arrest in such units. The majority of patients with coronary thrombosis, however, are admitted to general medical beds. The results of the treatment of cardiac arrest after myocardial infarction in general medical wards have been uniformly poor—Nachlas and Miller (1965) reported a 5% survival-rate and McNicol (1966) reported success in 10% of cases. In a review of attempted resuscitation in over 200 patients, Stemmler (1965) found a survival-rate of 7·2%.

The object of this report is to indicate that with adequate nursing instruction and a highly mobile resuscitation team the chance of successful treatment, outside an intensive-care unit, of cardiac arrest in patients with ischæmic heart-disease, should be reasonably good.

SUMMARY

The value of intensive-care units in reducing the mortality from cardiac arrest after myocardial infarction has been substantiated. But their role is limited by the fact that most patients who develop cardiac arrest after myocardial infarction do so before they have reached such units. A highly mobile resuscitation team, operating over a wide area within the confines of a large general hospital, will save approximately a third of patients who have a cardiac arrest after myocardial infarction. Since the majority of deaths from cardiac arrest happen immediately after the onset of infarction, a mobile resuscitation team should be able to reach the patient in his own home.

Requests for reprints should be addressed to Dr. J. S. Geddes, Royal Victoria Hospital, Grosvenor Road, Belfast 12.

Figure 3.3
Lancet 1966; 1:807-808

References

1. Eisenberg M. Bernard Lown and defibrillation. Resuscitation 2006;69:171-3.
2. Wiggers CJ. The physiologic basis for cardiac resuscitation from ventricular fibrillation – method for serial defibrillation. Am Heart J 1940;40:413-22.
3. Baskett TF, Baskett PJF. Frank Pantridge and mobile coronary care. Resuscitation 2001;48:99-104.
4. Pantridge JF, Geddes JS. Cardiac arrest after myocardial infarction. Lancet 1966;1:807-8.
5. Nachlas MM, Miller DI. Closed-chest cardiac resuscitation in patients with acute myocardial infarction. Am Heart J 1965;69:448-59.
6. Stemmler EJ. Cardiac resuscitation. A 1 year study of patients resuscitated within a university hospital. Ann Int Med 1965;63:613-8.
7. McNichol MW. The intensive care of patients with myocardial infarction. Practitioner 1966;196:209-14.

Chapter 4

Origins of the cardiac ambulance in Belfast

In the summer of 1964, as a new second year resident committed to a career in cardiology, John Geddes was invited by Dr Pantridge to spearhead the development of hospital-based cardiac resuscitation services. One aspect of Geddes' planned academic development was his desire to work towards a doctorate degree at the university, and he found this new field attractive as a subject for writing a thesis toward an MD degree. With this in mind, Geddes spent available periods of his limited spare time at the hospital library, reviewing the literature relevant to cardiac resuscitation. During a visit to the library in the spring of 1965 he came across a paper by Wallace Yater et al addressing the timing of coronary deaths among young American servicemen.[1] The key finding in this paper was that 60% of those who died from acute myocardial infarction did so within one hour of the onset of symptoms. Geddes informed Dr Pantridge of these findings whilst having a cup of afternoon tea in the ward clinical room. Pantridge instantly appreciated the significance and said: *'Well if that is so, that is what is happening in Belfast and we are just seeing the tip of the iceberg. We must go out and get these people.'* [2]

Further review of the literature, along with local experience (later published), confirmed the findings of the Yater group. In Seattle, in the late 1950s, Bainton and Peterson found that 63% of deaths occurred within one hour of the initial symptoms of myocardial infarction.[3] For comparison with these two reports, Mittra, working in Belfast on an unrelated study of myocardial infarction, found that the average time from symptoms to admission in the Royal Victoria Hospital (RVH) was twelve hours.[4]

McNeilly and Pemberton, also in Belfast, carried out an epidemiological study – the results of which were available to Pantridge and Geddes pre-publication. They reviewed 998 fatal cases of coronary artery disease occurring over twelve months in 1965-66, and found that 60% died before reaching hospital.[5] They expressed this carnage in dramatic terms: *'Those who are admitted to hospital represent, in fact, the survivors of a storm that has already taken its main toll.'* [5] Of the 479 who died before admission to hospital, and in whom the time interval was determined, 229 (48%) survived more than thirty minutes from the onset of symptoms. Published in 1968, two years after the cardiac ambulance was started in Belfast, this study gave impetus and further support to the principle of mobile coronary care. As McNeilly and Pemberton wrote, after noting that 48% survived more than thirty minutes: *'It is among these that there would appear to be special scope for the cardiac ambulance, providing that medical aid is sought and the ambulance is summoned without delay.'* [5]

The review of these data in July 1965 confirmed Pantridge's opinion that, while in-hospital CCUs had their place they could never cause a serious reduction in the overall mortality from myocardial infarction, when more than half of the deaths occurred before reaching hospital. Thus, faced with this high early mortality, due mainly to ventricular fibrillation – a correctable arrhythmia if treated promptly – Pantridge decided to create a system of pre-hospital mobile coronary care, based at the RVH.

When Frank Pantridge declared, *'We must go out and get these people,'* he had precedents to follow in the medical arena. In his autobiography, he compared the plight of the victim of a coronary attack to that of the battle casualties in the 18th century and noted the revolutionary approach taken by Napoleon's French army surgeon, Dominique-Jean Larrey (1766-1842).[6] Larrey found that soldiers wounded in battle took about twenty-four hours to reach the surgeons, who were set up some two miles behind the front lines. Upon arrival at the surgical unit most of the soldiers were dead or moribund. Larrey set up a lightweight 'flying ambulance' and transported surgeons and equipment to the battle area, where early intervention – mostly in the form of limb amputation – reduced the mortality.[7] Closer to home, looking from the back balcony of his wards across the intervening tennis courts and lawn, Pantridge could see the Royal Maternity Hospital where, in 1943, the Obstetric 'Flying Squad' had been established.[8] In the mid 1960s some 20% of women in Belfast delivered their babies at home under the care of district midwives and general practitioners (GP). When an acute complication arose, not unknown in obstetrics, the GP or midwife called the maternity unit and activated the flying squad. The obstetric registrar (senior resident), a midwife and a medical student gathered the packs containing instruments for delivery and operative obstetric procedures, including two units (in those days bottles) of O negative blood. They met the ambulance at the front of the maternity hospital and departed for the patient's home with suitable siren noises en route. The ambulance came from the depot in the hospital grounds and was not otherwise specially equipped for obstetrics. The problem facing Pantridge and Geddes was that they required a specially equipped ambulance modified to act solely as a mobile cardiac monitoring and resuscitation vehicle. To achieve this they would need an ambulance housed in the hospital grounds for immediate accessibility, capable of carrying a doctor and nurse in addition to the patient, and with all the equipment and drugs normally found in a CCU.

Since the primary objective would be the prevention of patient deaths due to ventricular fibrillation wherever it occurred, it would be essential that a DC defibrillator capable of being operated from batteries be carried in the ambulance. The defibrillator could of course be transferred to the patient's home and plugged into the house electrical outlets to correct ventricular fibrillation if it occurred there. A means of converting DC power derived from car batteries to 220 volts AC at 50 cycles per second (the standard of the United Kingdom power grid), with sufficient power output to charge the defibrillator multiple times would also be needed, and the appropriate device for this purpose was subsequently found to be a Static Invertor. A designated group of drivers for the cardiac ambulance would be selected from the staff of the Ambulance Depot, already situated in the hospital grounds.

Funding

Dr. Pantridge arranged a meeting with the members of the Northern Ireland Hospitals Authority at their headquarters in central Belfast in July 1965 and, in view of his major involvement in the data on which the proposal was based, Geddes was invited to attend.

Dr. Pantridge first described the success achieved with the operation of a mobile resuscitation system operating within the confines of the hospital and then drew attention to the numerically much greater problem of coronary deaths occurring in the community during the early period after the onset of a heart attack, where no sophisticated form of medical assistance was at hand. The great majority of these early deaths were likely to be the direct result of the eminently correctable rhythm disturbance of ventricular fibrillation. Next, he presented the available information regarding the feasibility of performing defibrillation outside hospital by means of a special ambulance carrying a portable defibrillator charged from a battery, and operated by trained personnel including a junior doctor and a nurse drawn from the staff of the cardiology wards of the Royal Victoria Hospital. In the mid 1960s it was still usual in the British Isles for people who suddenly became ill to contact their family doctor first, rather than to use the '999' system to call an emergency ambulance to transport them to hospital.

In 1965 there were some 100,000 people living within a one mile radius of the RVH. If the GP could reach the patient quickly, there would be a reasonable chance that the physician would arrive before cardiac arrest occurred, or at least in time to provide CPR and have a message transmitted to a special telephone number allocated for summoning the 'cardiac ambulance'. Further, if the symptoms initially described over the telephone were convincing and the GP was unable to come directly, it would still be possible for them to activate the special ambulance based at the hospital by telephone, and then travel to the scene as soon as possible.

While the members of the Authority were impressed by the information presented regarding the successful management of cardiac arrests within the hospital, they expressed doubts about the feasibility of reaching many of the patients situated in the community in time - especially if cardiac arrest were to occur shortly after the onset of symptoms. In rebuttal, Pantridge pointed out that the dismal status quo would continue unless the successful in-hospital resuscitation service was extended to the community. The members' final decision was that they would agree to fund the proposed scheme for one year, after which the situation would be reviewed. They were not, however, prepared to provide all of the necessary money. The physicians would have to apply for funding for the special ambulance and for the salaries of the dedicated junior doctor and of the one additional ambulance driver who would be needed. Fortunately, a subsequent application by Dr. Pantridge to the British Heart Foundation provided a grant of £2000 – enough to cover the salaries of the doctor and the driver for one year. After the first year Pantridge went to the Hospitals Authority to seek sustained funding for the mobile coronary care service. Apparently their attitude was quite negative until, as he later wrote, '....*it was pointed out that they might be held responsible for the deaths of coronary victims who perished because the unit was not available.*'[9] The funding was restored.

Having quickly grasped the practical logistics of early coronary deaths, and having identified what he saw as the solution, Pantridge pressed on rapidly – the cardiac ambulance was in service within six months. Pantridge provided the authoritative clout to convince the Hospitals Authority and secure funding, but it was left to Geddes (by now a third year resident) to carry the main organisational load of putting principle into action. To achieve this within six months was exceptional; imagine trying to accomplish this within the modern multilayered matrix of hospital administration.

Modification of the ambulance

Fortuitously, a large and powerful Daimler ambulance, which was several years old and destined for the scrap heap, was fully serviced and made available at the Ambulance Depot situated in the hospital grounds.

This vehicle had a powerful engine and was a little larger in size than the ambulance in common use at the time. In designing the interior lay-out of the special ambulance, it was essential that the stretcher should occupy the central area in order to permit access by the staff from the head end and from both sides. The doctor would sit at the patient's right side near the front, with a shelf to hold an ECG machine and the defibrillator, with other emergency equipment extending towards the back of the ambulance. In 1966, no battery-operated oscilloscope was available: however, the fact that long strips of the patient's ECG were obligatorily recorded on paper during transport meant that a more complete permanent record of the patient's cardiac rhythm was available for inspection afterwards. This helped facilitate audit and research. The accompanying nurse would sit at the patient's left side, with an area holding routine resuscitation equipment towards the front and a space for a suitcase holding emergency drugs behind. At the front end of the interior there was a spare seat on either side, and between these seats was a narrow space giving access to the driver's cab. Oxygen cylinders were stored on the nurse's side at the front.[10] (Figure 4.1)

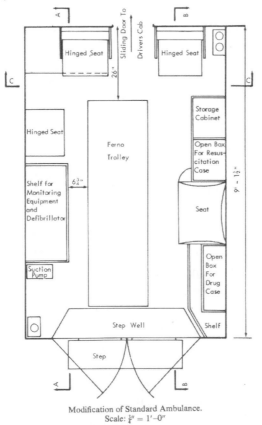

Modification of Standard Ambulance.
Scale: $\frac{3}{4}'' = 1'-0''$

Figures 4.1 Layout of cardiac ambulance (Ref 10)

Charging the defibrillator from car batteries

It was at first unclear how this could be achieved with a twelve volt car battery, even though this had the capacity to deliver quite a heavy current when needed. Fortunately, Alfred Mawhinney, the RVH cardiology technician, discovered that charging the defibrillator from a battery could be achieved with a piece of equipment known as a 'Static Invertor'. This device was commonly used to run high voltage electrical equipment, normally powered by an alternating current source, from lead acid batteries. A Static Invertor was purchased from Ulster X-Ray, the company in Belfast which normally supplied radiological equipment to the hospital. Shortly after it arrived Mawhinney connected it to a fully charged twelve volt battery and attached the defibrillator to the output side. When the latter was switched on and set to the maximum 400 Joule setting, the needle on the defibrillator dial immediately began to move up the scale from zero, leading to optimistic noises from those present. However, the rate of charging slowed and the energy level only reached about 150 Joules before charging ceased completely. There was also a smell of burning: the insulation on the connecting wires had melted as a result of the heavy current required for the Invertor. The trial was halted for that day. A few days later the experiment was repeated with a larger audience present. Two car batteries, connected in series (to provide twenty-four volts), were now attached to the Static Invertor using much thicker wires, which would not be expected to overheat, and the defibrillator was again connected to the output side of the Invertor. The defibrillator was switched on and on this occasion it charged quickly to 400 Joules without any overheating of the connecting wires; loud cheering ensued from the assembled throng.

Education of the General Practitioners

In the early autumn of 1965 Pantridge and Geddes began a series of ten o'clock Sunday morning classes for the general practitioners of the city. The aim was to provide training in CPR and inform them of the rationale and role of a mobile coronary care ambulance.The classes were held in the large lecture theatre known as 'The Old Surgical Extern' at the Royal Victoria Hospital. A CPR teaching mannequin was made available. The doctors, in groups of 10-15, were taught the need to avoid delay, either in reaching the patient, or in summoning the special ambulance if they believed that myocardial infarction was a possibility. They were not to feel embarrassed or fear retribution if their diagnosis turned out to be incorrect. The importance of prompt pain relief with morphine accompanied by an anti-emetic, together with reassurance of the patient while waiting for the mobile unit to arrive were emphasised. It was possible that such treatment might reduce the risk of life-threatening arrhythmias through a decrease in the production of adrenaline. The family doctors showed obvious interest in the new service, and in the possibility of preventing unnecessary deaths.

Liaison with the Ambulance Depot

Fortunately, the Ambulance Depot was in the hospital grounds and in October 1965, Pantridge and Geddes met with Mr. Bulger, the head of the Ambulance department. Among the items discussed was the need for a suitable driver and the avoidance of delay in the cardiac ambulance reaching the pick-up point for the staff at the junction of Musson Road and the Consultants' carpark - about 500 metres from the depot and just behind Wards 5 and 6. After the meeting, on the short drive from the depot back to the hospital (involving one ninety-degree bend and two others of forty-five degrees each), Pantridge went into Formula One mode, dropped into third gear and pressed the accelerator to the floor. On arrival at the planned pick-up point for the medical staff he stopped the car, looked at his watch and said *'That was exactly forty seconds.'* This would become the standard that ambulance drivers were expected to match: less than one minute from the call to arrival at the staff pick-up point. It also required reasonable fitness of the involved nurses and doctors, running an obstacle course from the ward, down stairs and around the tennis courts to the pick-up point. The increase in staff fitness was regarded as an appropriate plus in a cardiac unit. (Figure 4.2)

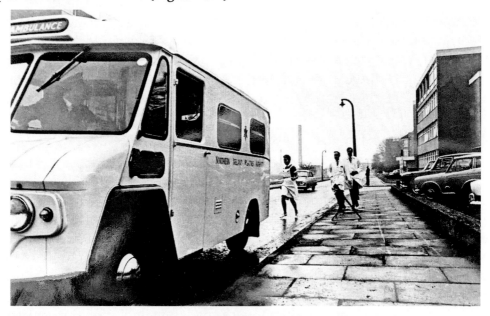

Figure 4.2 Staff Nurse, Geddes and Medical Student run to the cardiac ambulance at the RVH pick-up point.

A 'Trial Run'

One afternoon in October, well before the service was due to begin, Dr. Pantridge received a telephone call from a general practitioner who was seeing a patient not very far from the hospital. The patient, a male aged about sixty years, was feeling unwell and had a pulse rate of about forty per minute; the presumptive diagnosis was complete (atrio-ventricular) heart block. Pantridge immediately seized the opportunity to perform a 'trial run' with an ambulance carrying staff from the Cardiac Department and the chance to provide vital assistance to an ailing patient. He arranged with the Ambulance Depot for a standard ambulance to be made available, and told Geddes to find a nurse from Wards 5 and 6 to accompany him, bringing a sterile 'cut-down set,' local anaesthetic and a sterile pacing electrode, along with an ECG machine and an external pacemaker of the type frequently used in the ward.

The required items were quickly assembled, and Geddes, together with one of the staff nurses, met the ambulance at the designated pick-up point. They soon arrived with the patient to find the situation very much as originally described; an ECG confirmed atrio-ventricular block. Geddes performed a 'cut-down' under local anaesthesia and inserted the pacing electrode into a vein near the patient's left elbow. There had been reports in the medical literature of the successful insertion of pacemaker electrodes without the help of X-rays to guide the tip into the appropriate place in the heart. Geddes tried for several minutes to manipulate the tip of the electrode wire 'blindly' into the right ventricle, where pacing might be achieved, but without success. The arm was therefore covered with a sterile dressing and the patient carefully moved to the hospital, where he was taken straight to the cardiac catheterisation laboratory and the electrode easily manipulated into the right ventricle under X-ray control. Successful pacing was achieved, with normalisation of the heart rate, and the patient subsequently received appropriate long-term management.

Final preparations

During the days and weeks before the new service was scheduled to open on 1st January 1966, the medical and nursing staff who would be involved had ample opportunities to inspect the ambulance and its contents and make any last-minute suggestions. The special number of the red telephone (2-44-44) which would enable GPs to call the mobile unit (colloquially the 'Cardiac Ambulance'), was allocated at the main desk in Wards 5 and 6. 'Beepers' (pagers) were made available for the registrar and staff nurse on call, as well as the duty house physician.

Telephone numbers of the more senior doctors, available to provide advice from home in the evenings and at weekends, were posted in the ward (at a later date these individuals, too, were provided with 'long-distance' Beepers). A roster of the doctors on call for the cardiac ambulance was clearly displayed beside the red phone in Wards 5 and 6, as were the names and numbers of senior registrars (in addition to Dr. George Patterson, who ran the Cardiac Catheterisation Laboratory), who would provide so-called 'home cover' back-up. These physicians would come to the hospital to insert temporary pacemaker electrodes or perform other emergency procedures when indicated. Dr. Pantridge himself did not participate formally in the rota system but, when available, he was always prepared to provide advice.

Bearing in mind that the eyes of the members of the Northern Ireland Hospitals Authority, and others, would be trained on the efficiency of operation, and to facilitate audit, a logbook was kept in the unit to record the following times in each case: receipt of call, boarding the ambulance, arrival and departure of the ambulance at the patient's address, arrival in the Casualty department and admission of the patient to the cardiology ward.

Seen from half a century later, the 'Cardiac Ambulance', might be considered as a much larger version of an 'emergency cart', but capable of carrying trained staff in addition to emergency equipment over relatively long distances to the scene of a cardiac emergency. Having provided the necessary emergency treatment 'at the scene', it would be incumbent on the staff to ensure that patients were stable before attempting to transfer them to the hospital, 'without haste or fuss'. (Figure 4.3)

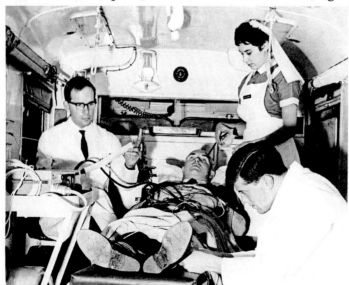

Figure 4.3

Staff Nurse, Geddes and Medical Student transfer patient from house to the ambulance.

Another requirement for the ambulance staff was to cope with a potential idiosyncrasy involving the plug on the defibrillator. This could cause difficulties if there was a need to plug in the defibrillator to the main electric supply in the patient's home. Several years earlier the power plugs in the United Kingdom as a whole, which had previously been manufactured in separate '5' and '15' Ampere sizes (unfused), with round 'prongs' (of a unique size and spacing for each size), were standardised to a single '13 Ampere' size with rectangular prongs and fitted with a fuse. In 1966 many houses still had the old five and fifteen Ampere rounded sockets. A special adapter was required, and made available in the ambulance, to connect the defibrillator to these old electrical sockets should it be necessary.

The adaptor, did not need to be used often, but an unexpected problem with it was to emerge during one emergency in an upstairs bedroom of a house in Belfast, several months after the mobile unit was launched. The patient went into ventricular fibrillation and Geddes and the nurse initiated CPR, while the two medical students were quickly dispatched to fetch the defibrillator from the ambulance. The adaptor was needed but shattered upon attempted insertion into the old electrical wall fitting. Geddes instructed the students to each hold a bare wire into one of the two 'active' wall sockets. Fortunately the defibrillator worked, the patient was successfully restored to sinus rhythm, and survived; neither student was harmed in this triumphant cardioversion!

1st January, 1966:
The launch of mobile coronary care

The doctor and nurse on duty were prepared for the first call from the Red Phone, but the hours passed and the team got on with their clinical duties on the wards. Each morning Dr. Pantridge came into the Wards 5 and 6 clinical room and asked expectantly, 'Well, any action last night?' Geddes had to provide the disappointing answer, 'No,' on six consecutive mornings. But at 5:20 p.m. on 6th January, 1966, the first call came through on the red telephone. Geddes took the call: earlier that day, a woman had developed severe chest pain and was now complaining of shortness of breath. To Geddes it was a clear-cut case for the cardiac ambulance, and together with the nurse on call ran downstairs and out to the road to board the cardiac ambulance, which had been alerted and was on its way from the depot. The team travelled at speed to the patient's home where the woman was in some distress. The ECG was recorded and showed evidence of an acute coronary attack affecting what appeared to be a relatively small area on the lateral wall of the heart. The family doctor, who was present, had already given her a pain-relieving injection

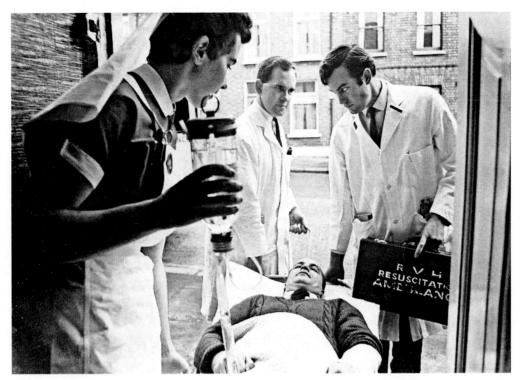

Figure 4.4
Geddes, Staff Nurse and Medical Student settle the patient into the cardiac ambulance before transfer to the hospital CCU.

and a diuretic, as there was evidence of mild heart failure. The patient, now comfortable, was carried to the waiting ambulance and transported without fuss to the RVH coronary care unit accompanied by her husband, Geddes and the nurse. (Figure 4.4) The usual tests confirmed that she had a lateral myocardial infarction. In due course she was discharged feeling well. This first call for the cardiac ambulance represented the initiation of Mobile Coronary Care. Although this call occurred at a time when both the nurse and the ambulance driver were shortly to go off duty, they, together with Geddes felt a sense of great satisfaction that the first call had been successful.

The Cardiac Ambulance, which became better known as 'The Mobile Coronary Care Unit', was now fully 'launched'. January 1966 would be remembered as the beginning of a new era in the management of the acute coronary attack, and ultimately in the development of expanded pre-hospital emergency medical services.[11]

Initial results with the 'cardiac ambulance'

Between its inception on 1st January 1966 and 31st March 1967 the results obtained with the Mobile Coronary Care Unit were collected with a view to publication,[11] and for possible presentation at the annual meeting of the Association of Physicians of Great Britain and Ireland, which it so happened was to be held in Belfast at the Queens University Clinical Institute, adjacent to the Royal Victoria Hospital, in the spring of that year.

Following the 'slow' beginning in early January, 1966, there had been a progressive increase in the frequency of calls for the mobile unit as the year advanced. Some streamlining of the system to ensure there were no avoidable delays in picking up the medical team at the defined rendezvous point was performed. Otherwise everything ran smoothly and almost 80% of the patients were reached within fifteen minutes of receipt of the call.

During the unit's first fifteen months of operation, there were 338 calls resulting in the admission of 312 patients suspected of having acute myocardial infarction. One hundred and fifty-five (50%) of the 312 had clear-cut electrocardiographic evidence of acute myocardial infarction, and another 96 (31%) had prolonged chest pain without definite evidence of infarction. Twenty-eight (9%) had a normal electrocardiogram despite prolonged chest pain: in twenty-two (7%) the pain was considered not due to myocardial ischaemia, and in the remaining eleven cases (3%) the call was judged to have been unjustified.[11] (Figure 4.5)

Seventy-eight of the 155 patients with clear-cut infarction came under intensive care within two and a half hours of symptom onset and one hundred and one within four hours. During the entire period in hospital twenty-one of the patients admitted via the mobile unit developed ventricular fibrillation, of whom fifteen were resuscitated successfully and ten of these were long term survivors. The mortality among patients with definite infarction was 20%. It was considered probable that this high figure reflected the selection of relatively severe cases for transport via the mobile unit by the referring general practitioners during the early part of the project.

Ten patients were resuscitated from ventricular fibrillation outside hospital. In all ten, fibrillation developed within four hours of symptom onset and the circulation was re-established following defibrillation, although only six survived to be discharged from hospital. Details regarding the four who did not survive are set out below:

A seventy-five year old woman (the first to be resuscitated before reaching the hospital, in June, 1966) developed ventricular fibrillation in the ambulance and was defibrillated by the house physician, but unfortunately she died of rapidly progressive congestive heart failure two hours after admission.

58

The Lancet · Saturday 5 August 1967

A MOBILE INTENSIVE-CARE UNIT IN THE MANAGEMENT OF MYOCARDIAL INFARCTION

J. F. PANTRIDGE
M.C., M.D. Belf., F.R.C.P.
PHYSICIAN-IN-CHARGE

J. S. GEDDES
M.D., B.Sc. Belf.
REGISTRAR

CARDIAC DEPARTMENT, ROYAL VICTORIA HOSPITAL, BELFAST 12

Summary The risk of death from myocardial infarction is greatest in the twelve-hour period after the onset of symptoms. Despite this, the hospital admission of a large proportion of patients is delayed for more than twelve hours, and many die in transit to hospital. A scheme has been described involving the use of a highly mobile unit which enables intensive care to reach the patient when he is at most risk. The unit has been used in the transfer of patients to hospital. No death has occurred in transit in a fifteen-month period. Ten examples of successful resuscitation outside hospital are reported. 5 of these patients are now alive and well. Thus it has been shown perhaps for the first time that the correction of cardiac arrest outside hospital is a practicable proposition.

Figure 4.5
Lancet paper 1967;2:271.

A fifty-five year old man collapsed at a dance hall and it was unclear what initial resuscitative efforts had been made by the attendant: ventricular fibrillation was removed by the registrar and the man was transported to the hospital, he failed to regain consciousness and died of cerebral damage several days later.

A forty-two year old woman complaining of chest discomfort developed ventricular fibrillation at home in the presence of her family doctor, who performed CPR while awaiting arrival of the ambulance. Sinus rhythm was established with some difficulty. Eventually she became stable enough to be moved, but she did not re-awaken and died within the next few days.

A forty-nine year old man, who might easily have died of his life-threatening cardiac arrhythmia at his home, and for whom the full range of electrical therapies available on the Mobile Coronary Care Unit were utilised, was particularly unfortunate not to become a long-term survivor. On the afternoon of 21st November, 1966, Geddes was recording the patient's ECG at his home when ventricular fibrillation appeared. Defibrillation was easily achieved, but the rhythm was now high grade atrioventricular block with a conspicuously slow ventricular rate, and the systolic blood pressure was only 30 mm of mercury. A bipolar pacing electrode (brought from the ambulance) was promptly introduced into a left-sided vein under local anaesthesia, and advanced into the central circulation. Fortunately, the electrode tip immediately entered the right ventricle and, with the external pacemaker switched on at a rate of seventy per minute, ventricular pacing at the same rate became evident on the monitor. The blood pressure immediately returned to a normal level, and finally the electrode was attached to the skin with a suture to prevent accidental displacement. He was then carefully moved to the ambulance and brought to the hospital coronary care unit. While in the coronary care unit his condition remained satisfactory, and his problem with atrioventricular conduction resolved within two days. The pacing electrode was removed some days later. Because he was regarded as having had a fairly large amount of cardiac damage at the time of his heart attack, and because he was having relatively frequent ventricular 'ectopic' heart beats (regarded as a 'warning sign' of an ongoing risk of recurrent ventricular fibrillation) he was kept in hospital for a full three-week period after his admission and commenced on one of the 'anti-arrhythmic' drugs then in use, probably Procainamide. Tragically, there was a recurrence of ventricular fibrillation within twenty-four hours of his planned discharge and, on this occasion, resuscitation was unsuccessful.

This last case illustrates what was technically possible in 1966 regarding effective electrical treatments for the control and correction of life-threatening disturbances of cardiac rhythm. It also shows the sparsity of information then available for determining the individual risk of dangerous ventricular arrhythmias among patients recovering from heart attacks, especially when a relatively large amount of myocardium had been damaged.

Presentation of the results to the Association of Physicians of Great Britain and Ireland

Geddes presented the results to the Association meeting, held in April 1967 at a lecture theatre in the Clinical Institute adjoining the RVH. His was the first presentation of the one-day meeting. He had been warned by Dr. Pantridge that it was unlikely the applause from the audience would be very loud. There was in fact an uproar of dissent. The main complaint by the physicians present was that the operation of the Mobile Unit departed from the basic tenet relating to the management of the patient with a recent heart attack, which should be to maintain calm, relieve pain and only when conditions were stable would it be appropriate to move the patient as smoothly as possible to the hospital. It was quite wrong to 'bundle the patients into hospital', as Dr. Geddes was proposing! Geddes replied that the whole objective of the mobile unit was, as he had already stated, to achieve exactly what the speaker was proposing - but to no avail. Dr. Pantridge reassured Geddes when the session ended that 'most of these doctors have spent last night on the Liverpool-Belfast boat crossing the Irish Sea and didn't get a wink of sleep, so they acted like a swarm of angry bees when they heard your presentation.'

Several members of the junior staff made substantial contributions to the running of the unit, and/or to research, during the first and the subsequent several years. Memorable among these were: Jennifer Adgey, Desmond Allen, Don Keegan, Basil McNamee, Conor Mulholland, Norman Patton, Michael Scott, Fred Stanford and Samuel Webb.

Long-term follow up of resuscitated patients

The first follow-up study was published in the Lancet in 1967, immediately following the report of the results obtained with the Mobile Coronary Care Unit during its initial fifteen months of operation.[12] The objective of this publication was to demonstrate that prolonged survival following resuscitation from ventricular fibrillation complicating an episode of acute myocardial ischaemia or infarction was possible, and could indeed become commonplace. The patients reported were the first fifty survivors of ventricular fibrillation managed at the Royal Victoria Hospital: forty-seven of them had a recent myocardial infarction, the remaining three had definite evidence of ischaemic heart disease. Seventeen of the patients had had more than one cardiac arrest, with eight of these having experienced three or more episodes (maximum thirty-three). The majority were prescribed procainamide for their long term antiarrhythmic therapy.

Ten of the patients died from a cardiac cause within twenty-two months after discharge from hospital and four of these deaths were attributed to a recurrent cardiac arrest. In three of the four, the fatal cardiac arrest occurred between two and three months after the initial resuscitation (one possibly related to discontinuation of an anti-arrhythmic drug). It is of interest that, at the time when this paper was written, three patients who had originally survived between ten and thirty-three episodes of ventricular fibrillation had been followed for periods of six to twenty-one months without experiencing any recurrence of their arrhythmia.

The status of thirty-one of the fifty patients was considered to be clinically mild prior to cardiac arrest and that of the remaining nineteen (with evidence of pulmonary congestion or reduced peripheral circulation) was classed as severe. The estimated two-year survival for the mild group was 85%, and that for the whole series 55%.

A longer follow-up study was published in 1971 and represented 160 patients (79% male) who had been admitted to the Royal Victoria Hospital between 1964 and 1969 and who had a final diagnosis of either acute myocardial infarction (151), or of acute coronary insufficiency with an abnormal electrocardiogram (9).[13] All of the patients studied were survivors of ventricular fibrillation which occurred during their index admissions. One half of the entire group were considered clinically to be in mild condition, with another 30% showing signs of moderate circulatory embarrassment and the remaining 20% having 'considerable' cardiac failure. All of the patients had at least one episode of ventricular fibrillation, 20% of the episodes having occurred outside hospital, 20% while in the Coronary Care Unit and 60% in general medical wards. The most important finding of this study was that those patients who survived ventricular fibrillation occurring within four hours of symptom onset had a better survival rate at thirty-six months (78%) in comparison with those in whom fibrillation developed later (52%). The former group was on average younger than the latter and the majority had experienced a mild coronary attack. The majority of the survivors of ventricular fibrillation complicating a relatively severe attack had developed cardiac arrest more than four hours after onset. It is also of interest that, in five of six patients who survived multiple (and sometimes very numerous) episodes of ventricular fibrillation, the first episode of arrhythmia occurred twelve or more days after onset of the original symptoms.

During the time of these follow-up studies no means were available to determine global and regional left ventricular function non-invasively, and radio-nuclide myocardial perfusion scans aimed at detecting areas of heart muscle supplied by narrowed or occluded arteries had yet to be developed. The widespread availability of coronary angiography to delineate these arteries in detail was still some years away. The outlook of some of these 'post-fibrillation' patients might have been improved by the selective administration of a beta-sympathetic blocking agent in conservative dosage, but the evidence in favour of this approach was not yet available.

References

1. Yater WM, Traum AH, Brown WG et al. Coronary artery disease in men eighteen to thirty-nine years of age. Report of 866 cases, 450 with necropsy examinations. Am Heart J 1948;36:334-72, 481-526, 688-722.
2. Eisenberg MS. Life in the Balance. New York: Oxford University Press;1997.p208-17.
3. Bainton CR, Peterson DR. Deaths from coronary heart disease in persons fifty years of age and younger. N Engl Med J 1963;152:1090-3.
4. Mittra B. Potassium, glucose and insulin in treatment of myocardial infarction. Lancet 1965;2:607-9.
5. McNeilly RH, Pemberton J. Duration of last attack in 998 fatal cases of coronary artery disease and its relation to possible cardiac resuscitation. BMJ 1968;3:139-42.
6. Pantridge JF. An Unquiet Life: Memories of a Physician and Cardiologist. Antrim: Greystone Books; 1989.p85-6.
7. Baker D, Cazoloa JB, Carli P. Larrey and Percy – a tale of two Barons. Resuscitation 2005;66:259-61.
8. Gibson ED, Ritchie JWK, Armstrong MJ. The changing role of the obstetric flying squad. Ulster Med J 1980;49:126-30.
9. Pantridge JF, Wilson C. A history of prehospital coronary care. Ulster Med J 1996;65:68-73.
10. Pantridge JF, Adgey AAJ, Geddes JS, Webb SW. The Acute Coronary Attack. Tunbridge Wells: Pitman Medical Publishing;1975.p127.
11. Pantridge JF, Geddes JS. A mobile intensive care unit in the management of myocardial infarction. Lancet 1967;2:271-3.
12. Geddes JS, Adgey AAJ and Pantridge JF. Prognosis after recovery from ventricular fibrillation complicating ischaemic heart disease. Lancet 1967;1:273-5.
13. McNamee BT, Robinson TJ, Adgey AAJ, Scott ME, Geddes JS and Pantridge JF. Long-term prognosis following ventricular fibrillation in acute ischaemic heart disease. BMJ 1971;4:204-6.

Chapter 5

Limitation of myocardial damage: 'tissue is time, time is tissue'

The initial raison d'etre of the mobile coronary care unit was simply to prevent or correct ventricular fibrillation and other potentially life-threatening arrhythmias, relieve chest pain and dyspnoea, and to provide efficient and calm transfer to hospital. The three fundamental principles of initial treatment in the early days of mobile care included:

- Administration of oxygen.
- Relief of pain by the intravenous administration of narcotic (usually morphine).
- Cultivating a calm and unhurried environment, especially during removal from the scene and in transit by ambulance.

However, Pantridge and Geddes encountered a whole array of unanticipated phenomena during the acute phase of myocardial infarction, which were largely due to inappropriate activation of one or both branches of the autonomic nervous system.[1] Their observations and research laid the foundation for much of the progress in the treatment of acute myocardial infarction over the last fifty years.

Autonomic disturbances complicating the acute coronary episode – significance and treatment

It had been noticed by those staffing the Mobile Coronary Care Unit that, among patients with myocardial infarction seen relatively soon after the onset of symptoms, the heart rate and blood pressure could be either relatively low or relatively high. Geddes had, in fact, encountered a patient with unexplained bradycardia and an unusually low blood pressure within a few months of the operation of the mobile unit, and had corrected the problem empirically with a modest dose of atropine. Discussion of this case with Dr. Pantridge prompted a detailed prospective study of these 'autonomic disturbances' associated with acute myocardial infarction.[2] As more patients were seen by the team, pulse rates above or below the normal 60-100 per minute were encountered, and abnormal blood pressures were observed in the same direction as the pulse. Samuel Webb became a registrar in Cardiology in 1968 and took an interest in the meticulous collection of data. Recording the data relating to the occurrence of the autonomic disturbances presented a particular challenge because the deviations in rate could appear unpredictably at any moment, and at that time invasive recording of arterial pressure was impracticable while the patient was in transit in the ambulance. In addition, even a minor invasive procedure might result in an alteration in the data obtained. Fortunately, the electrocardiograph which had been installed in the mobile unit in 1966 was still in service, and for the formal study the recording paper was run continuously, with clock time calibrations added, and the periodic blood pressure readings were inscribed upon it.

The group reported its findings in seventy-four patients (seventy-two under the age of seventy) who were reached by the cardiac ambulance within thirty minutes of the onset of acute myocardial infarction.[3] There were signs of autonomic disturbance in sixty-eight of the seventy-four (92%): vagal overactivity was apparent in forty-one (55%) and sympathetic overactivity in twenty-seven (37%), with 'unmasking' of sympathetic overactivity in a further seven following atropine. Careful atropine administration, however, often resulted in a smaller and more acceptable increase in rate.

Among eight patients with complete atrio-ventricular block who were given atropine, conduction rapidly improved in five with restoration of normal blood pressure but in a sixth patient hypotension persisted, and in two others atropine had no effect on conduction. Patients showing evidence of sympathetic overactivity were treated with the beta-blocking agent practolol given intravenously, resulting in a reduction in heart rate associated with a decrease in the degree of ST segment elevation.[2,3]

The overall mortality among patients aged under seventy was 9.7%. This figure was remarkably low in comparison with a mortality in the region of 20% or higher expected for an otherwise comparable group of patients not seen and treated early after the onset of symptoms. It was reasonable to conclude that the correction of abnormalities of heart rate and blood pressure had resulted in the salvage of at least some myocardial tissue at the margins of the developing infarct – supporting the 'time is tissue' concept.

Geddes spent the year, June 1969 to June 1970, in Salt Lake City, Utah, pursuing a project in experimental Electrophysiology with Professor Abildskov at the University of Utah.[4] In May, 1970, Dr. Pantridge paid a three-day visit to Geddes at Salt Lake. Over dinner on the first evening, Pantridge announced with a gleam in his eye that the current mortality rate of patients in his wards with a diagnosis of myocardial infarction, who were admitted via the Mobile Unit, was as low as 9% (in contrast to rates prior to the advent of mobile care, in the region of 20% or more). The critical combination of therapies likely to be responsible for this reduction was the relief of pain prior to transport and the prompt correction of the autonomic disturbances. Such interventions would remove the wastage of available oxygen in the myocardium resulting from tachycardia and hypertension, and improve the delivery of oxygen either by increasing the perfusion pressure or by lengthening the duration of diastole.

Shortly before he left Salt Lake City, Geddes was contacted by Dr. Stanley Sarnoff (1917-1990), the developer of the auto-injector. He proposed the self-use of automatic atropine injectors (the AtroPen, designed for use by the military in the event of chemical warfare) for the purpose of preventing or correcting possible reflex bradycardia resulting from occlusion of the right coronary artery. This injector could be used by individuals experiencing symptoms suggestive of acute myocardial infarction when they were isolated from medical help. Geddes felt that, although the effect of the atropine administered could be salutary if the person already had, or was about to develop bradycardia with hypotension, the drug could be very harmful if the anterior descending branch of the left coronary artery were occluded, and he therefore did not recommend it. Interestingly enough, Dr. Sarnoff later founded a company, Survival Technology, Inc. for the further design and introduction of auto-injectors, filing in 1988 to patent an auto-injector adapted for the self-administration of tPA (tissue plasminogen activator) for patients with symptoms consistent with acute myocardial infarction.[5]

The advent of the beta-adrenergic blocking drugs (propranolol in 1965, and later - in 1969 - the cardio-selective agent metoprolol) would make a significant but not decisive addition to the armamentarium. More than another decade would elapse before a reasonably accurate means of determining the individual risk of life-threatening arrhythmia occurring late following apparent recovery from a myocardial infarction, and the effect of therapy on that risk, would be developed.

Thrombolysis

Despite the undoubted benefits derived from correction of the autonomic disturbances associated with the acute phase of myocardial infarction, the stenosis or occlusion of the coronary artery which had precipitated the acute heart attack would not be altered by the administration of atropine or a beta-blocking agent. Although coronary arterial occlusion is a complex process, it is usual for the final event to be the formation of a thrombus within the residual lumen of the artery. Based on this assumption, the search began in the sixties for methods of preventing the propagation of the clot or, once it formed, 'dissolving' it in order to preserve myocardial tissue. The decades following would provide a deeper understanding not only of the metabolism and biochemistry of clot formation in coronary disease but also of approaches to attacking the problem.

In the spring of 1979 Geddes attended a lecture delivered by Hewan Dewar (1913-2012), Cardiologist at the Royal Victoria Infirmary, Newcastle-upon-Tyne, on the possibility of reopening occluded coronary arteries. Dewar presented his experience in the management of a patient who had developed what must have been a paradoxical embolus (originating in the systemic veins) to the right coronary artery, which had broken into two or three fragments and was causing chest discomfort. He had treated the patient with an intravenous infusion of streptokinase which had succeeded in reopening the artery and relieving the pain.[6,7]

The era of coronary thrombolysis employing streptokinase or one of its derivatives took root in the U.K.[7] During the early 1980s Geddes had the opportunity, on a few occasions, to try out a more sophisticated preparation given by intravenous injection, with good results - including dramatic relief of chest discomfort and 'freezing' of the infarction process on the ECG, associated with almost visible collapse of the initially elevated ST segment.

The dawn of the 21st century shone a light on both pharmacological and mechanical methods of restoring the patency of coronary vessels compromised by clot. Almost all of these approaches to restoring patency, 'reperfusion' as it came to be known, would depend heavily on the development of a structured system which revolutionised the approach to the early treatment of acute myocardial infarction, and that system would depend heavily on the provision of high-quality, evidence-driven pre-hospital care systems which were only in their infancy in the sixties.[8,9,10] (see Chapter 10)

Angioplasty

In 1977, the first coronary angioplasty procedure for an occluded vessel was performed in Zurich, Switzerland, by a German radiologist, Andreas Gruentzig (1939-1983), who had developed the technology for opening occluded coronary arteries by means of balloon angioplasty.[11] Subsequently, in 1980, Gruentzig emigrated to the USA and became a faculty member in medicine and radiology at Emory University in Atlanta. Following Gruenzig's arrival at Emory, the opening of occluded arteries became a routine procedure for the cardiac catheterisation laboratory, with the advantage that the opening of the artery could be more predictable and more nearly complete, and the infarction process (at least temporarily) halted.[12]

In time, the immediate insertion of rigid stents into the opened arteries became routine in order to avoid an unacceptable rate of post-procedure occlusion.[13] Anti-thrombotic agents are given as a routine after angioplasty in order to minimise the risk of rethrombosis.

In 2017 the lesson, *"tissue is time, time is tissue"* has been well and truly learned.

References

1. Adgey AAJ, Geddes JS, Mulholland HC, Keegan DAJ, Pantridge JF. Incidence, significance and management of early bradyarrhythmia complicating acute myocardial infarction. Lancet 1968;ii:1097-99.
2. Pantridge JF, Adgey AAJ, Geddes JS, Webb SW. The Acute Coronary Attack. Pitman Medical Publishing; Tunbridge Wells: 1975.p26-78.
3. Webb SW, Adgey AAJ, Pantridge JF. Autonomic disturbance at onset of acute myocardial infarction. BMJ 1972;3:89-92.
4. Geddes JS, Burgess MJ, Millar K, Abildskov JA. Accelerated repolarization as a factor in re-entry simulation of the electrophysiology of acute myocardial infarction. Am Heart J 1971;88:61-8.
5. Sarnoff S. Automatic injector for emergency treatment. Survival Technology, Inc. Bethesda, MD; US4795433, 1989.
6. Dewar HA, Stephenson P, Horler AR, Cassells-Smith AJ, Ellis PA. Fibrinolytic therapy of coronary thrombosis: controlled trial of 75 cases. BMJ. 1963;1:915-20.
7. Sikri N, Bardia A. A history of streptokinase use in acute myocardial infarction. Tex Heart J. 2007;34:318-27.
8. Nallamothu BK, Krumholz HM, KO DT, LaBresh KA, Rathore S, Roe MT et al. Development of systems of care for ST-elevation myocardial infarction patients: gaps, barriers and implications. Circulation. 2007;116:e68-e72.

9. Le May MR, So DY, Dionne R, Glover CA, Froeschl MPV, Wells GA, et al. A citywide protocol for primary PCI in ST-segment elevation myocardial infarction. N Engl J Med. 2008;358:321-40.

10. Bata A, Rehman Quraishi AU, Love M, Title L, Beydoun H, Lee T, et al. Initial experience with pre-activation of the cardiac catheterization lab and emergency room bypass for patients with ST-elevation myocardial infarction in Halifax, Nova Scotia. Internat J Cardiol. 2016;222:645-47.

11. Barton M, Gruentzig J, Hussmann M, Rosch J. Balloon angioplasty-the legacy of Andreas Gruentzig. Frontiers Cardiovasc Med. 2014;1(15):1-25.

12. King SB. The development of interventional cardiology. J Am Coll Cardiol. 1998;31(suppl2):64B-88B.

13. Sigwart U, Puel J, Mirkovitch V, Joffre F, Kappenberger L. Intravascular stents to prevent occlusion and restenosis after transluminal angioplasty. N Engl J Med. 1987;316:701-6.

Chapter 6

Development of pre-hospital coronary care outside Belfast

Pantridge and Geddes published their initial results on mobile coronary care in the 5th August 1967 edition of the Lancet.[1] Some three months before, on 19th May 1967, they had presented these results to the Association of Physicians of Great Britain and Ireland which happened to meet in Belfast. They received a cool reception and, as Pantridge was later to describe, *'We were disbelieved and indeed, to some extent ridiculed. The unfavourable comments emphasised the lack of need for pre-hospital coronary care, the prohibitive costs and the dangers of moving a patient who had a recent coronary attack.'* [2] This negative response from the British physicians of influence was disappointing, but did not dent the enthusiasm of Pantridge and Geddes.

Some fifty kilometres north of Belfast lies the town of Ballymena and its Waveney Hospital, which had established a coronary care unit (CCU) in November 1964. The consultant physician, Robert Kernohan, following the Belfast example, and in consultation with them, had started a mobile coronary care ambulance along similar lines in late 1966. This served a rural population of about 165,000 and three smaller district hospitals that did not have CCUs. In 1968 they reported six months experience with 164 calls.[3] Even in this rural area, the average time between the call and provision of intensive care was less than thirty minutes. Three of five patients with ventricular fibrillation were successfully resuscitated at home, and survived to leave hospital.

At the Ulster Hospital, which served east Belfast and was remote from the ambulance depot, a different type of service was established in 1969.[4] A small van was set up with the appropriate medical equipment, including a defibrillator. The local general practitioners (GPs) were informed of the service and, upon their call to a special line in the hospital's CCU, a doctor and nurse from the unit drove the van to the site of the call. Resuscitation and stabilisation of the patient were undertaken as needed, and if required an ordinary ambulance was summoned to transport the patient to the hospital. The doctor or nurse accompanied the patient and the other drove the van back to the hospital. In the first fifty calls the mean time from call to attendance at the patient was twelve minutes: one person was successfully defibrillated at home and subsequently discharged from hospital.[4]

The Irish Heart Foundation organised a mobile coronary care service for the city of Dublin coordinated with the five city hospitals that had CCUs. This was the first pre-hospital coronary care system to use specially trained ambulance personnel (before the term 'paramedic' was widely adopted). The service started in December 1967 and they reported a three year experience in 1971.[5] Twenty patients had cardiac arrest at the place of collapse (ten) or during transport in the ambulance (ten). Of these seventeen were successfully resuscitated and defibrillated by the ambulance crew and eleven (55%) survived. The Dublin system had an on-call doctor available to be summoned by the ambulance team, but this was only used in 1.6% of calls. They concluded, *'In light of this experience the routine employment of doctors may be unnecessary and involve an uneconomical use of special skills.'*[5]

Throughout Great Britain, in contrast to Ireland, the attitude toward pre-hospital coronary care generally ranged from disinterest to dismissive. In September 1967, Pantridge presented his results to an international meeting on coronary care in Edinburgh. Once again his work was challenged and one Edinburgh cardiologist quoted the French General Maréchal Bosquet's famous comment on the suicidal charge of the Light Brigade in the Crimea: *'C'est magnifique, mais ce n'est pas la guerre.'* [2,6]

In that same month of September 1967 a different attitude was shown in the United States in an article in *Time* magazine entitled *'Immediate Counterattack.'* This described the limitations of hospital CCUs, if up to one quarter of affected patients died before admission. The option of rushing the necessary equipment, including a defibrillator, to the patient to forestall these early deaths was discussed. The article declared *'There is just one place in the world where this is being done, Northern Ireland's dour capital city of Belfast.'* (Pantridge, while welcoming the positive review, always resented the description of Belfast as 'dour'). The *Time* item also suggested that the presence of a defibrillator in the White House would be appropriate, in view of the past history of myocardial infarction in the sitting President (Lyndon Johnston). As it turned out this was a prescient observation (see later).

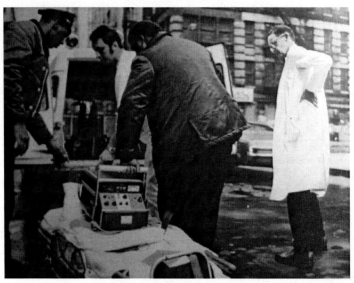

Fig 6.1 William Grace (1916-1977), on right, supervising the loading of the New York cardiac ambulance.

William Grace, a cardiologist at St Vincent's Hospital, New York City was the first physician to visit Belfast with a view to replicating the mobile coronary care unit in New York.(Figure 6.1) Shortly after the Lancet article was published he spent ten days in Belfast, participated in rounds on Wards 5 and 6 at the RVH and accompanied John Geddes in the cardiac ambulance on a number of calls. Upon return to New York he established the first mobile coronary care ambulance in the United States. The medical and nursing personnel left the hospital within five minutes of receipt of a 'cardiac' call. In his report of the first 161 cases Grace confirmed the high incidence (52/161) of arrhythmias. There were three cases of ventricular fibrillation treated in the community, with one long term survivor.[7] Grace was also influential in establishing 'Life Support Stations' with resuscitation equipment, ECG monitoring, and defibrillators. These were set up where large numbers of people congregated, such as factories, office buildings, sports stadia and transportation centres.[8]

In the late 1960s, in the United States, it was estimated there were about 400,000 deaths from acute myocardial infarction per year (>1000/ day)[9], and that about two-thirds of these died before reaching hospital.[10] These figures, plus the fact that many had 'hearts to good to die,' were the impetus to reproduce the Belfast approach of pre-hospital coronary care.[11] Obstacles were a lack of physicians to staff the ambulance and the fact that the existing rescue ambulance services were often under the control of local Fire or Police departments. In the early 1960s, in many communities

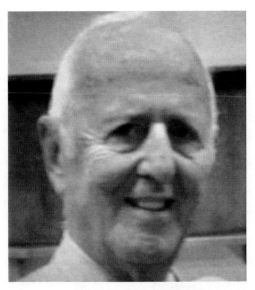

Fig 6.2 Eugene Nagel

in North America, the ambulance service was run by morticians.[12] Many of the fire chiefs were keen for their personnel to learn and adopt basic CPR, but often baulked at their members being entrusted with more advanced skills such as defibrillation, intubation and intravenous drug administration.

In Miami, Eugene Nagel, an anaesthetist with an interest in CPR, took a different approach.(Figure 6.2) Working with the Miami Fire Department he pioneered the use of ECG telemetry, with a central unit providing guidance to the fire crew.[13] Once he had the telemetric data to prove the need for defibrillation and drug administration he was able to convince the fire chief and city commissioners of the rationale for and feasibility of training the fire crew in advanced skills. He proceeded to provide special training for nine selected members of the fire department – now referred to as emergency medical technicians or paramedics. In dramatic fashion he had them demonstrate their practical skills in front of the fire chief and a group of the city commissioners: this included all nine, in turn, intubating Nagel under topical anaesthesia.[14] Thus he was ultimately able to provide the full complement of resuscitation services with paramedic personnel: CPR, ECG telemetry, defibrillation, intravenous access and drug administration – all with remote physician advice.[15]

Leonard Cobb, a cardiologist in Seattle, also spent some days in Belfast at the Pantridge unit.(Figure 6.3) Working through the Seattle Fire Department he took a more comprehensive approach. In March 1970 he implemented a 'two tiered response' in which the existing fire department's

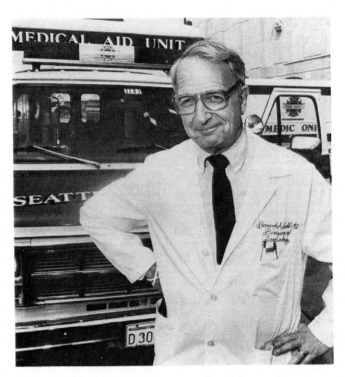

Fig 6.3 Leonard Cobb

first response units provided CPR, followed by a mobile coronary care unit staffed by specially trained paramedics for ECG interpretation, defibrillation, intubation and intravenous drug administration if necessary. The coronary care ambulance was, in fact, a modified mobile home and was known as 'Medic One'; less complimentary monikers were 'Moby Pig' and the 'Wonder Bread Van.'[16] For the first nine months a physician accompanied the unit, but thereafter the paramedics operated alone. During the first year the Medic One unit resuscitated sixty-one patients of whom thirty-one were ultimately discharged from hospital.[17] In 1972 Cobb added a third level to his tiered response – training citizens to do CPR. In the world's first such programme the aim was to train 100,000 people in Seattle, and after twenty years more than 500,000 local citizens had completed CPR training.[16]

In 1969 Richard Crampton took up his appointment as director of the CCU in Charlottesville, at the University of Virginia, having trained as a resident in New York. (Figure 6.4) The year before, he had read and been intrigued by the work of Pantridge and Geddes. Thus, during one of his family's annual visits to his wife's parents in Kilkenny, he took a side trip to Belfast and rode the cardiac ambulance. In March 1971 he was able to establish a mobile cardiac care system with both physicians

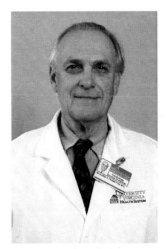

Fig 6.4 Richard Crampton

and paramedics, closely modeled on the Belfast unit.[18,19] At a later visit to Virginia, Pantridge was told by the locals, with some pride, of their first 'life-save.' It involved a prominent local horse trainer who collapsed in a pile of manure at a major horse show. After eight bouts of defibrillation he recovered completely. Pantridge's response was that he hoped the man had his tetanus shot.[18] Considerable publicity descended upon Crampton in April 1972 when former President Lyndon Johnson had a myocardial infarction while visiting his daughter in Charlottesville.[20] The President was treated by Crampton using the Pantridge system and recovered.

Thus by the late 1960s / early 1970s, in addition to those outlined above, mobile coronary care units had been set up in many cities or regions of the United States including Columbus, Ohio,[21] Portland, Oregon[22] and Los Angeles,[23] among others.[24] In Portland a fortuitous sequence of events added early credibility to the mobile coronary care unit. The mayor of Portland, who approved the system, and the owner of the ambulance company which ran the system, both collapsed on separate occasions and were successfully resuscitated and defibrillated by the ambulance paramedics.[18] Similar pre-hospital coronary care schemes were established in Perth and Sydney, Australia.[25,26] Indeed, in their 1975 book *The Acute Coronary Attack*, Pantridge and his group noted forty-five mobile coronary care units in thirteen countries: twenty-four of which were in the United States.[27]

Notwithstanding the initial negative response of the medical/cardiological establishment in Britain, there were isolated pockets of innovation. Small mobile coronary units, often with very limited resources, sprang up in Newcastle,[28] Salford,[29] Barnsley,[30] Dudley,[31] Brighton[32] and

Bristol.[33] Most of these services were set up by the drive and enthusiasm of individuals rather than by institutions.

Douglas Chamberlain, a cardiologist in Brighton, was stimulated to start a mobile cardiac ambulance by a chance encounter during a home consultation. The patient had a cardiac arrest during his examination, Chamberlain started CPR, and told the man's wife to dial 999 and summon the ambulance. When the ambulance eventually arrived the defibrillator, which required two men to lift, exploded and caught fire. Chamberlain felt '…..we ought to be able to do better.' [34] He therefore organised one of the first mobile coronary ambulance services staffed by specially trained paramedical personnel.[32]

In some units a more pragmatic approach was taken to include all cases needing emergency care – not just cardiac patients. In Bristol, Peter Baskett, an anaesthetist who had worked with Dr Pantridge as a student and house physician, started a mobile resuscitation ambulance '..for all patients requiring resuscitation regardless of the underlying disease or injury.' [33] The specially equipped vehicle was staffed by ambulance personnel trained in the provision of analgesia,[35] intravenous access, intubation and defibrillation – backed in selected cases, by anaesthetists.[36] Some two-thirds of the calls were for trauma or cardiac care, with an even split between motor vehicle accidents and coronary cases. The estimated cost of a life 'definitely saved' was £250.[33]

In Moscow, there was a tradition of a physician-staffed ambulance being summoned to the scene by the first response emergency team, if a cardiac case was encountered.[37] However, as Pantridge was to discover on a visit to Moscow in 1970, as part of a World Health Organisation consultant team, they had no defibrillator in the 'heart' ambulance. Thus, Pantridge felt '….. the whole point of a mobile unit had been missed.' [2]

In 1975 a Joint Working Party was set up by the Royal College of Physicians and the British Cardiac Society to consider the care of patients with coronary heart disease.[38] Among other things they recommended that the Department of Health and Social Security (DHSS) in the United Kingdom 'actively encourage the development of mobile coronary care.' [39] The DHSS, however, was advised by a Standing Medical Advisory Committee (SMAC), the members of which decided that the case for mobile coronary care had not yet been made. Despite other evidence, they accepted the findings of two reports from Nottingham and the West of England.[40,41] Unfortunately, both of these studies were poorly designed and omitted many patients in the early phase of myocardial infarction – the very ones who would benefit from early mobile coronary care. Thus, the conclusion of a lack of benefit was an unwitting bias built into these studies.[42]

It was to be seven more years, in 1982, before SMAC accepted the recommendations of the Working Party. As the 1980s progressed the National Health Service ambulance system was equipped with defibrillators and operated by trained paramedic personnel.[42]

The ' life saves' gained from pre-hospital defibrillation in patients with myocardial infarction were impressive and, of course, dramatic. However, for the sceptics, and as the Belfast group put it, *'The true benefit of coronary care can only be appreciated by recording its effect on the case fatality rate within a defined community.'*[43] Such a reduction was recorded by Crampton in Virginia[44] and Sherman in Illinois.[45] However, this was at a time of decline in the overall death rate from ischaemic heart disease throughout the United States.[46,47] The Belfast and Ballymena groups approached this with a classic study of two geographically and demographically similar towns in Northern Ireland: Ballymena and Omagh.[48] The hospitals of both towns had a CCU, but only Ballymena had a mobile coronary care ambulance. Over the fifteen-month study period the community mortality from myocardial infarction at twenty-eight days was statistically lower in Ballymena (40%) compared to Omagh (59%).[48] One-third of the improved outcome was realised in the first hour after the onset of symptoms and attributable to the prevention of arrhythmic death. The remaining two-thirds of the better outcome was deemed due to the beneficial effect of early treatment limiting myocardial damage (see chapter 5).

References

1. Pantridge JF, Geddes J S. A mobile intensive care unit in the management of myocardial infarction. Lancet 1967;2:271-3.
2. Pantridge JF. An Unquiet Life. Antrim: Greystone Books; 1989.pp88, 93-4.
3. Kernohan RJ, McGucken RB. Mobile intensive care in myocardial infarction. BMJ 1968;3:178-80.
4. Barber JM, Boyle D, Chaturvedi NC et al. Mobile coronary care. Lancet 1970;2:133-4.
5. Gearty GF, Hickey N, Bourke GJ, Mulcahy R. Pre-hospital coronary care service. BMJ 1971;3:33-5.
6. Julian D. Frank's legacy from a European perspective. Ulster Med J 2010;79 (Suppl 1):7-9.
7. Grace WJ, Chadbourn JA. The mobile coronary care unit. Dis Chest 1969;55:452-5.
8. Grace WJ. Prehospital care and transport in acute myocardial infarction. Chest 1973;63:469-72.

9. Provisional Statistics, Annual Summary for the United States, 1969. National Center for Health Statistics, Public Health Service, US Dept Health, Education, and Welfare, 1970.

10. Fulton M, Julian DG, Oliver MF. Sudden death in myocardial infarction. Circulation 1969;40(Suppl 4) :182-93.

11. Beck CS, Leighninger DS. Death after a clean bill of health. JAMA 1960;174:133-5.

12. Howard JM. Historical background to 'Accidental death and disability': the neglected disease of modern society. J Prehospital Emerg Care 2000;4:285-9.

13. Nagel EL, Hirschman JC, Mayer PW, Dennis F. Telemetry of physiologic data: An aid to fire-rescue personnel in a metropolitan area. Southern Med J 1968;61:598-62.

14. Eisenberg MS. Eugene Nagel and the Miami paramedic program. Resuscitation 2003;56:243-6.

15. Nagel EL, Hirschman JC, Nussenfeld SR et al. Telemetry – medical command in coronary and other mobile emergency care systems. JAMA 1970;214:332-8.

16. Eisenberg MS. Leonard Cobb and Medic One. Resuscitation 2002;54:5-9.

17. Cobb LA, Conn RD, Sampson WD. Pre-hospital coronary care: the role of a rapid response mobile intensive coronary care system. Circulation 1971;44(Suppl 11):11-45

18. Crampton RS. Frank's legacy from a North American perspective. Ulster Med J 2010;79(Suppl 1):4-6.

19. Crampton RS, Stillerman R, Gascho JA et al. Prehospital coronary care in Charlottesville and Albermarle County. Virginia Med Monthly 1972;99:1191-4.

20. New York Times. 11 April 1972. p28.

21. Warren JV, Mattingly C, Rand S. The design and operation of a mobile coronary care unit. Circulation 1969;40, Suppl 111, 212-8.

22. Rose LB, Press E. Cardiac defibrillation by ambulance attendants. JAMA 1972;219:63-8.

23. Lewis AJ, Bebout C, Criley JM. Eighteen months experience with a mobile intensive care unit. Circulation 1971;44:, Suppl 11:192-7.

24. Eisenberg MS, Pantridge JF, Cobb LA, Geddes JS. The revolution and evolution of prehospital cardiac care. Arch Intern Med 1996;156:1611-19.

25. Robinson JS, McLean ACJ. Mobile coronary care. Med J Aust 1970;2:439-42.

26. O'Rourke MF et al. Modified coronary ambulance. Med J Aust 1972;1:875-8.

27. Pantridge JF, Adgey AAJ, Geddes JS, Webb SW. The Acute Coronary Attack. Tunbridge Wells: Pitman Medical Publishing;1975.p130-6.

28. Dewar HA, McCollum JPK, Floyd M. A year's experience with a mobile coronary resuscitation unit. BMJ 1969;4:226-9.

29. Rifkin FM. Pre-hospital coronary care service. BMJ 1971;3:310-11.

30. Sandler G, Pistevos A. Mobile coronary care: the coronary ambulance. Br Heart J 1972;34:1283-91.

31. Kubik MM, Bhowmick BK, Stokes T, Joshi M. Mobile cardiac unit: experience from a West Midland town. Br Heart J 1974;36:238-42.
32. White NM, Parker WS, Binning RA, Kimber ER, Ead HW, Chamberlain DA. Mobile coronary care provided by ambulance personnel. BMJ 1973;3:618-22.
33. Baskett PJF, Diamond AW, Cochrane DF. Urban mobile resuscitation: training and service. B J Anaesth 1976;48:377-85.
34. Baskett PJF. Douglas Chamberlain – a man for all decades of his time. Resuscitation 2007;72:344-9.
35. Baskett PJF, Withnell A. Use of entonox in the Ambulance Service. BMJ 1970;2:41-3.
36. Nolan J, Chamberlain D, Soar J, Parr M, Zorab J. Peter Baskett – 40 years as a resuscitation leader and mentor. Resuscitation 2008;77:279-82.
37. Moiseev SG. The experience of rendering first aid to myocardial infarction patients in Moscow. Sovetsk Med 1962;26:30.
38. McDonald L. Mobile coronary care – yesterday and today. In: Geddes JS (ed). The Management of the Acute Coronary Attack. London: Academic Press;1986.p77-83.
39. The Royal College of Physicians of London and the British Cardiac Society. The care of the patient with coronary heart disease: report of a joint working party. JR Coll Phys Lond 1975;10:5-46.
40. Mather HG, Pearson NG, Read KLQ et al. Acute myocardial infarction: home and hospital treatment. BMJ 1971;3:334-8.
41. Hill JD, Hampton JR, Mitchell JRA. A randomised trial of home-versus-hospital management for patients with suspected myocardial infarction. Lancet 1978;1:837-41.
42. Acheson D. DHSS attitude to mobile coronary care. In: Geddes JS (ed). The Management of the Acute Coronary Attack. London: Academic Press;1986. p85-91.
43. Wilson C. Effect of a medically-manned coronary care unit on community mortality. In: The Management of the Acute Coronary Attack. Geddes JS(ed). London: Academic Press;1986.p39-50.
44. Crampton RS, Aldrich RF, Gascho JA et al. Reduction of prehospital, ambulance and community death rates by the community – wide emergency cardiac care system. Am J Med 1975;58:151-65.
45. Sherman MA. Mobile intensive care units: an evaluation of effectiveness. JAMA 1979;241:1899-1901.
46. Cooper R, Stamler J, Dyer A, Garside D. The decline in mortality from coronary heart disease, USA 1968-1975. J Chronic Dis 1978;31:709-20.
47. Stern MP. The recent decline in ischemic heart disease mortality. Ann Intern Med 1979;91:630-40.
48. Matheson ZM, McCloskey BG, Evans AE, Russell EJ, Wilson C. Mobile coronary care and community mortality from myocardial infarction. Lancet 1985;1:441-4.

Chapter 7

Evolution of Defibrillation

By the early 1960s the evolution of defibrillators in the United States had culminated in a radical change away from the very large, unwieldy and excessively heavy machines of the 1950s (which had delivered alternating current shocks of a strength in the region of 700 volts), to the still large, 'Lown' direct current defibrillator (see Chapter 2), which provided shocks measuring, in terms of energy content, up to a maximum of 400 Joules (volts times amperes), to be discharged through the patient's chest over a period of several milliseconds. In practical terms, the energy required to achieve defibrillation could now be provided in a manner which had been shown to achieve high efficacy, and which would eliminate the risk that appreciable heating of the tissues (including the heart), might occur.

The bulk and weight of the early cardioverter-defibrillator (Lown) available in 1963 were partially attributable to the inclusion of the synchroniser and the monitor within its outer casing, as described in Chapter 2. A smaller version of this defibrillator, with the oscilloscope and synchroniser omitted, and weighing only 25kg (55 lb), became available a year later and was purchased for the Royal Victoria Hospital cardiology ward in late 1964. This was quite suitable for the emergency correction of ventricular fibrillation appearing on a cardiac monitor or electro-car-diographic recording (with the external recording device momentarily disconnected during administration of the shock). However, the use of this smaller machine in the case of a perfusing arrhythmia (e.g. ventricular tachycardia, atrial fibrillation) risked precipitating ventricular fibrillation, should the shock coincide with the 'vulnerable period' of a spontaneous QRS complex.[2]

Early efforts to design a portable defibrillator at Johns Hopkins in Baltimore were progressing in the laboratory of Drs. Kouwenhoven, Knickerbocker and Jude and represented the natural extension of their defibrillation research which, by serendipity, produced the modern form of closed-chest cardiac massage announced by them in 1960.[3] Their 'portable' defibrillator, developed by Claude Haggard in 1961, although weighing over 20 kg. (45 lbs.), was indeed independent of mains (house) current, operated with two forty-five volt batteries and was contained in a plastic carrying case.[4,5] It was developed to be carried by Electric Company trucks to help resuscitate linemen who suffered electric shocks. There is no record of its use in practice.

At the RVH the electrocardiographic monitoring equipment in the Coronary Care Unit was initially serviced (and from time to time upgraded, first to provide a magnetic tape in a fifteen minute recording loop and, later, electronic signal storage) by an outside company. However, during 1965, Dr. Pantridge became increasingly preoccupied with the need to establish an electronics laboratory in the hospital, dedicated to the needs of the Cardiology Department. Already, one of the hospital technicians, Mr. Alfred Mawhinney, had shown great aptitude and enthusiasm for performing repairs and for dealing with the outside equipment suppliers.

The creation of a dedicated Cardiology Electronics Laboratory was agreed in principle towards the end of the year and the position of Chief Technician to assist in running it was advertised. There was only a small number of applicants for the position, but by far the most impressive among them was a Mr. John Anderson, who at that time was working for Shorts, a company which developed and manufactured aircraft in Belfast. He was duly appointed and took up his position at the hospital on 1st January, 1966, rapidly acquiring a grasp of the needs, and service requirements of the monitoring and defibrillation equipment, of the Coronary Care Unit, the Resuscitation Service and the Mobile Coronary Care Unit.

Important as these developments were, John Anderson's primary mission, as seen by Dr. Pantridge, was the development of a truly portable defibrillator of a radically reduced weight in comparison with the original Lown Cardioverter. The weight of the capacitor and the associated components (inductor coil and choke) were of crucial importance in achieving this goal. Upon enquiry, Mr. Anderson ascertained that the only capacitors in existence which would fulfill the requirement for reliability and light weight were those employed by the United States National Aeronautics and Space Administration for their space programme (NASA). With Dr. Pantridge's assistance, in April, 1966, he formulated a letter to NASA requesting permission to acquire the vital capacitors; fortunately this was granted without delay. Minimising the size and weight of the defibrillator still presented a number of challenges, in particular the incorporation of a light-weight rechargeable battery capable of providing enough energy for a substantial number of shocks (maximum shock strength 400 joules, similar to the Lown machine) before a recharge became necessary, and the attachment of two separate 'paddles' with attached metal discs and

81

connecting cables for administering the shocks to the patient.

Fortunately, Dr. Pantridge himself hit on the brilliant idea of having only a single conventional external paddle, whilst placing the second metal disc on the underside of the defibrillator body itself (letting the all-important discharge button come within easy reach of the user's thumb). The final weight of the 'Pantridge Portable Defibrillator' was just under 3.2 kg. (7 lb) and the maximum stored energy was 400 Joules. It was powered by a 20.4 volt nickel-cadmium battery. The fifty micro-farad capacitor, charged to 4,000 volts and discharged through a fifty milli-Henry inductor to a fifty ohm load, resulted in a critically damped monophasic pulse of twelve milliseconds' duration. This configuration corresponded with that determined by Peleska to be optimal for the correction of experimentally induced ventricular fibrillation.[6] (Figure 7.1)

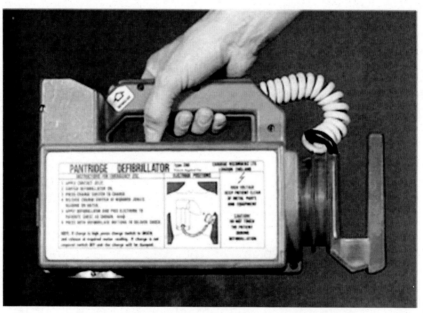

Figure 7.1 The Pantridge portable defibrillator

The Pantridge defibrillator was manufactured by Cardiac Recorders Ltd (London) and became available in 1974. In the same year, two articles by Tacker and colleagues from Houston, Texas, seemed to cast doubt on the premise that a maximum stored energy of 400 Joules was sufficient to terminate ventricular fibrillation in the great majority of patients.[7,8] A prospective trial of low energy defibrillation was initiated in Belfast in August, 1974, and during the subsequent five months forty-three patients were treated for eighty-two episodes of ventricular fibrillation.

Thirty-seven of the forty-three had suffered a recent myocardial infarction. A maximum of two low energy shocks of 200 Joules were administered for each episode before a higher energy was tried. Low energy defibrillation was successful in all but two patients, and appeared to be unrelated to patient weight - the successes included five patients who weighed in excess of 90 kg. Both of the patients in whom low energy defibrillation failed were given high energy shocks which removed the fibrillation, but a spontaneous circulation could not be restored in either.[9] The lower the energy of the shock from the defibrillator, the lower the risk of damage to the myocardium. Pantridge once said that 'he had created his defibrillator, not for personal gain or glory, but simply to save lives'.

Pre-hospital Coronary Care in the United States

The publication of the initial results obtained with the Belfast Mobile Coronary Care Unit generated much interest in prehospital coronary care amongst many physicians in the United States. In fact, there was already anecdotal evidence that some individual doctors had ventured outside the hospital environment in order to treat patients in a state of cardiac arrest with defibrillation. For example, Eugene Nagel in Miami had become aware of Pantridge's work in 1967 and during the following year Nagel started a programme for the training of fire-rescue squads in the use of defibrillators.[10] Medically-manned mobile units were set up by William Grace in New York (1969)[11] and by Richard Crampton in Charlottesville (1972).[12]

Paramedical/emergency medical technician units were established by Benson and Safar in Pittsburgh (1969),[13] Criley and Lewis in Los Angeles,[14] and by Leonard Cobb in Seattle (1970).[15] Many other units were established in other parts of the United States.[16] (See Chapter 6)

The Implantable Defibrillator

During the late 1970s there was growing awareness in medical circles that it would soon be possible to implant an automatic cardiac defibrillator in the human body. Michel Mirowski was developing an implantable defibrillator for use in patients who had recurrent potentially lethal cardiac arrhythmias resistant to drug therapy. It so happened that, following a medical meeting in Europe in March 1976, Drs. Mirowski and Pantridge found themselves on the same train travelling through Belgium to Amsterdam. They discussed an idea of Pantridge's that there should be an automatic externally worn defibrillator but, as Mirowski later told Geddes, he did not feel the idea was practicable. In 1978, Geddes visited Mirowski and his colleague, Morton Mower, at the Sinai Hospital in Baltimore, and saw the laboratory where Dr. Mirowski performed his developmental work on the implantable defibrillator. Fortuitously a dog with a defibrillator implant already in situ was walking freely in the laboratory, and Mirowski arranged for a demonstration of the function of the defibrillator on this animal. Mirowski's assistant held a radio transmitter briefly over the side of the dog's chest and about five seconds later the dog lost consciousness and fell to the floor. There followed a convulsive movement as the defibrillator delivered its shock and within seconds the dog looked around and jumped to its feet, eyeing Geddes with understandable suspicion.

During the remainder of the visit Mirowski, Mower and Geddes discussed the future of the project, and the first human defibrillator implant which they said was in the foreseeable future. The first procedure actually took place almost two years after Geddes' visit, at the Johns Hopkins Hospital.[17] The surgical team was led by Dr. Levi Watkins, the first black Chief Surgical Resident ever at that hospital,[18] assisted by Vivien Thomas, the renowned cardiovascular technician responsible for training surgical residents in the technique[19], with Dr. Mirowski in attendance. Today it is a routine procedure for patients who have life-threatening arrhythmias which cannot be reliably controlled by other means.

Recent Advances in External Defibrillators

The advantages of the Pantridge miniature external defibrillator have been extended considerably during the past forty years with the introduction of new features which enhance performance while keeping the size and weight of the defibrillator to a minimum. These features include:

1. *Impedance-compensation.* A high transthoracic impedance reduces the current and energy delivered, decreasing the probability of successful defibrillation. Kerber[20] introduced the concept of automatic measurement of transthoracic impedance prior to administering a defibrillatory shock, and adjusting the administered energy to provide a constantly high probability of successful defibrillation.

2. *Biphasic Defibrillation Waveform.* The original direct current defibrillators had either a completely monophasic waveform or a small negative 'tail' at the end of the shock. Biphasic waveforms with a more conspicuous terminal negative portion have been shown to improve greatly the probability of successful defibrillation, and modern defibrillators include this feature. A study published by Martens et al in 2001, compared an 'impedance-compensated'

biphasic exponential waveform with two slightly different 'monophasic' waveforms combined (one with a minimally negative 'tail').[21] This study included one hundred and fifteen patients who had out-of-hospital cardiac arrests due to ventricular fibrillation and were managed by the emergency medical services. It compared the results obtained with two varieties of shock delivered by automatic external defibrillators: biphasic or monophasic. The findings were: (1) the efficacy of biphasic shocks in correcting ventricular fibrillation was greater than that of monophasic shocks, and (2) the time intervals from the beginning of rhythm analysis to both the first shock and the first successful shock were shorter for the biphasic devices than for the monophasic devices. However, although more of the patients receiving biphasic shocks experienced a return of spontaneous circulation than did those given monophasic shocks, this difference was not statistically significant.[21] Nevertheless, the above findings supported the superiority of biphasic over monophasic defibrillation. Two other randomised studies produced similar results, with trends favouring biphasic shocks.

3. *Current-Based Defibrillation.* The term, 'shock energy' (measured in joules – volts multiplied by amperes of current) was originally employed as a convenient descriptor of the potential of an electrical discharge to terminate ventricular fibrillation. It is, however, the actual current flowing through the myocardium that determines whether or not conversion of fibrillation to another rhythm will result, and this in turn will be determined by the voltage applied to the chest and the electrical resistance of the intervening tissues. The term 'Active Impedance Compensation' was coined to convey the concept of automatic variation of the voltage applied to the chest in such a way that a predetermined current will flow through the myocardium. The process led to the coining of the term, 'Current-Based Defibrillation.' In pursuit of this principle, Gliner and colleagues performed a study in which the 'basal' energy of the shock was set at 150 Joules biphasic, and the actual current delivered was achieved by automatic adjustment of the voltage until the desired current was reached. In a study of one hundred consecutive victims of cardiac arrest, 97% of 450 episodes of ventricular fibrillation were corrected with no more than three biphasic shocks. The outcome of the attempted resuscitation was that an organised rhythm was present in 65%, while asystole and ventricular fibrillation were present in 25% and 10% respectively.[22]

4. *Enlargement of Defibrillator pad sizes.* Larger pads significantly reduce impedance and allow increased current flow for a given voltage. Special adhesive conductive pads began to be employed in place of 'paddles' for use with emergency defibrillators in the early 1980s. They were of a size comparable with the previously used paddles, in the region of 8 cm diameter, and they removed the necessity for a member of the resuscitation team to hold the paddle firmly against the patient's skin as had previously been the case. With the realisation that the electric current associated with the administered shocks is of critical importance to the success of defibrillation, the possibility that the reduced resistance associated with a larger pad size might facilitate defibrillation was explored by Dalzell et al in Belfast. Use of the larger pads more than doubled the success rate (82 vs 31% for a single shock, and 97 vs 46% when a second shock was given).[23]

Deployment of Defibrillators in Public Places

Since the 1990s, there had been a growing impetus for the deployment of automated defibrillators in public places to allow access by the general public, including railway stations, airline terminals, aircraft, sports stadia, etc. Success of this venture depended upon accuracy of rhythm detection, ease of use, and public awareness of the technique of cardiopulmonary resuscitation (CPR). In Brighton, England, Douglas Chamberlain dedicated much of his career to pioneering the use of resuscitation techniques.[24] In 1989 he set up a programme, with help from the British Heart Foundation, for the initiation of training for Transport Police at Brighton and Victoria (London) railway stations. As a result, during the two-year programme, five people were resuscitated from cardiac arrest who would otherwise have died. The National Defibrillator Programme was started in Britain in 2004.[25]

Defibrillators and Mobile Care in Rural Areas

For a discipline such as Mobile Coronary Care where speed is of the essence, there is an obvious inconsistency between the fundamental requirements and the practical impossibility of reaching ill patients at a long distance from the base hospital. The Belfast Cardiac Ambulance did, however, sometimes travel as far as twenty miles in order to transfer a patient who was potentially unstable from another hospital – whether from paroxysms of ventricular tachycardia, or from ventricular pauses secondary to atrioventricular block (if the source hospital was unable to provide facilities for temporary cardiac pacing).

For critically ill patients with heart attacks, however, it was clearly impractical for the hospital-based mobile coronary care unit, as originally designed, to venture far beyond the city limits. Attempts had to be made, however, to devise a system for dealing with cardiac emergencies occurring in rural areas. In the early 1970s such a system was developed by Peter Baskett in Bristol and Douglas Chamberlain in Brighton. They organised advanced training for ambulance personnel, who in turn became the first paramedics in Europe, and a profession in their own right. These paramedics used a mobile resuscitation unit which carried a defibrillator, and included equipment for transmitting electrocardiograms to the hospital.[24-27]

As will be outlined in Chapter 10, current mobile intensive care systems have been designed and have demonstrated success using collaborative designs with continuous remote and in-field physician supervision in partnership with highly-trained paramedical personnel.[28,29] Such systems include cadres of volunteer 'first responders' and the placement of automated external defibrillators (AED's) in sports clubs, arenas and mass gatherings of every kind- including rock concerts, casinos and even bingo halls.[30] (figure 7.2)

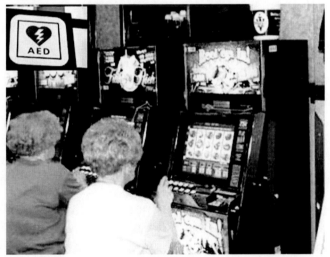

Figure 7.2 AED (Automated External Defibrillator). These are placed in areas with mass gatherings and where risk factors for myocardial infarction may be aggravated by the excitement of the moment

These growing regionalised systems of mobile coronary care, in some jurisdictions, reflect the structure of successful models of regionalised trauma care. In sparsely-settled regions in Canada, Australia and the United States combined ground-and-air systems with components of local community support for AED programmes are showing promise in respect to the outcomes of both cardiac and major trauma patients.

Defibrillators at Air Terminals and on Aircraft

Geddes spent a period of time (1996-7) in Sydney, Australia, working in conjunction with Dr. Michael O'Rourke and his staff studying Clinical Electrophysiology. He was invited to perform an audit of the results of a study being run by Eric Donaldson (medical director of Qantas Airlines) of the impact of cardiac defibrillators carried on board Qantas passenger aircraft on the outcome of cardiac arrest resulting from ventricular fibrillation. This study had been in progress for the previous sixty-five months and an article presenting the results was subsequently published in the journal *Circulation* in November, 1997.[31]

It was generally known that many lives were being lost each year due to cardiac arrest occurring on passenger aircraft and at airline terminals. In flight, each such episode necessitated diversion of the airplane to the nearest airport at significant expense, and the probability of survival of the passenger concerned was very poor. For the Australian airline Qantas the cost of these events was particularly high because of the considerable distance between recognised airports. In 1991, Semi-automatic External Defibrillators (AEDs) (Laerdal Heartstart 3000) were installed in the major international Australian Terminals and into each of the fifty-five international Qantas Boeing fleet. All the installations were completed by August 1992, and the Qantas staff was trained to operate the device and supervise the management of cardiac arrest. All cabin crew were trained in cardiopulmonary resuscitation with routine refresher training, which included extrication of unconscious passengers from their seats. The Qantas medical kit contained all the equipment needed for advanced life support (drugs to be administered by a physician volunteer). At the major terminals, a registered nurse was responsible for the dedicated AED.

During the five-and-a-half-year study period Qantas flew 203,191 flights and carried over thirty-one million passengers on its international flights. Over this period there were twenty-seven episodes of cardiac arrest on aircraft and nineteen at the major Australian international terminals. The AED was used in all of these episodes, and for monitoring purposes only on another sixty-three acutely ill persons (54 in aircraft and 9 in terminals). Of the twenty-seven episodes of in-flight cardiac arrest necessitating CPR and the use of the AED, six passengers (all with witnessed cardiac arrest) were in ventricular fibrillation (VF), successfully terminated in five, with one remaining in VF despite the application of eight shocks. All nineteen cardiac arrests in major Australian airport terminals were witnessed; VF was present in seventeen (89%), with four long-term survivors.[31]

Since this initial study both national and international airlines routinely carry AEDs as part of their onboard medical equipment and subsequent analysis of recent experience proves the practicability and successful outcome for many travelers who otherwise would be unlikely to survive the time taken to prepare for and execute an emergency landing.[32,33] Several modern emergency medical services systems include a specialised section of their communications centre designed to provide EMS physician advice to aircraft in flight for any flight crews caring for a passenger in distress.[34]

Summary and conclusions

Starting with the original 'Lown' defibrillator of the early 1960s which opened the door to practicable defibrillation, predominantly in the hospital environment, and the primitive monitoring equipment which accompanied it, the sophistication of the equipment steadily increased as the weight and size were reduced. Even before this process had become established, the first prehospital coronary care unit ('Cardiac Ambulance') with a 400 Joule defibrillator on board was launched in Belfast in1966. By March 1967, this mobile unit had proved its worth in terms of lives saved, in conjunction with the in-hospital coronary unit. Supported by an effective electronics laboratory, the way was open for further developments, culminating in the production of the world's first truly lightweight (3.2 kg) defibrillator of unique design and it was not long before the amount of energy required for successful defibrillation was shown to be no more than 200 Joules for most patients.

The development of the implantable defibrillator in 1980 marked another historic milestone. Patients who have recurring ventricular fibrillation despite maximal medical therapy now have an avenue which offers them the possibility of leading reasonably active lives. For patients in whom the automatic implantable defibrillator is impracticable an alternative is the wearable cardioverter-defibrillator (WCD) which is capable of performing the same defibrillation functions as the implantable version.

Refinements such as the discovery of the improvement in effectiveness associated with the use of biphasic defibrillation waveforms, impedance compensation and increased defibrillator pad sizes led to the possibility of producing even lighter weight defibrillators. The development of fibrillation detection circuitry opened the door to the use of miniature defibrillators by paramedical personnel outside the hospital environment, with a further increase in the saving of lives.

A major advance made possible by the above developments was the incorporation of miniature defibrillators in ambulances used in rural settings. These devices have even been carried by doctors in their cars. Paramedics quickly adopted defibrillators in the USA, and prehospital 'coronary' schemes came into operation there during the late sixties and early seventies. A major step forward included the introduction of semi-automatic defibrillators and later fully automated machines into passenger aircraft and airport terminals, thus enabling the correction of ventricular fibrillation wherever sudden collapse due to ventricular fibrillation was encountered. The research and work that enabled the Belfast group to reduce the size and weight of defibrillators fostered the development of even smaller devices and combined them with modern telecommunications unimagined in the 1970s. Clinical trials are underway, with several reported, of the feasibility and EMS system design of AEDs in rural areas delivered to the scene via 'unmanned aerial vehicles' (UAVs or 'drones').[35] (Figure 7.3)

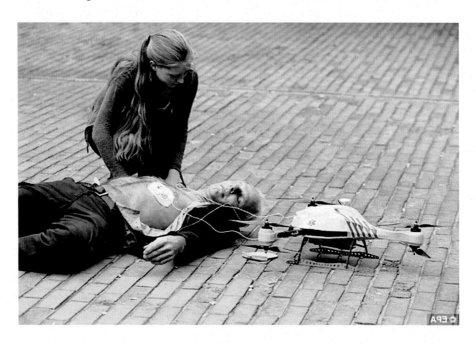

Figure 7.3 Unmanned Aerial Vehicles – 'Drones' – may take the place of static (fixed-place) AEDs in the future as research progresses to document response times and logistic challenges [35].

References

1. Akselrod H, Kroll M W, Orlov MV. History of defibrillation. In: Efimov IR, Kroll MW, Tchou, PJ, editors. Cardiac bioelectric therapy – mechanisms and practical implications. New York: Springer; 2009. p 15-40.
2. Wiggers CJ, Wegria R. Ventricular fibrillation due to single, localized induction and condenser shocks applied during the vulnerable phase of ventricular systole. Am J Physiol 1940;128:500-05.
3. Kouwenhouven WB, Jude JR, Knickerbocker GG. Closed-chest cardiac massage. JAMA. 1960;173:94-7.
4. White R. Shocking history: the first portable defibrillator. JEMS. 1995 Oct;41-45.
5. Beaudouin D. Reviving the body electric. Johns Hopkins Engineer. Fall 2002;27-32.
6. Peleska B. Optimal parameters of electrical impulses for defibrillation by condenser discharges. Circulation Research. 1966;18:10-7.
7. Tacker WA, McNamara, D, Guiliani, E, Geddes LA. An energy dose for human ventricular defibrillation (abstract). Am J Cardiol. 1974;33:172.
8. Tacker WA, Galioto FM, Guiliani E, Geddes LA. Energy dose for human trans-chest electrical defibrillation. N Engl J Med. 1974;290:214-15.
9. Pantridge JF, Adgey AAJ, Webb SW, Anderson J. Electrical requirements for ventricular defibrillation. BMJ.1975;2:313-5.
10. Nagel EL, Hirschman JC, Nussenfeld SR, Rankin D, Lundblad E. Telemetry-medical command in coronary and other mobile emergency care systems. JAMA. 1970;214:332-8.
11. Grace WJ, Chadbourn JA. The mobile coronary care unit. Chest. 1969;55:452-5.
12. Crampton RS, Stillerman R, Gascho JA, Aldrich RF, Hunter FP, Harris RH, et al. Prehospital coronary care in Charlottesville and Albemarle County. Va Med Monthly. 1972;99:1191-6.
13. Safar PJ. From Vienna to Pittsburgh for anesthesiology and acute medicine. In: Fink BR, McGoldrick KE, editors. Careers in anesthesiology; vol 5. Park Ridge, IL: Wood Library-Museum of Anesthesiology; 2000. p 204-212.
14. Lewis AJ, Ailshie G, Criley JM. Pre-hospital cardiac care in a paramedical mobile intensive care unit. Calif Med 1972;117:1-8.
15. Schaffer WA, Cobb LA. Recurrent ventricular fibrillation and modes of death in survivors of out-of-hospital ventricular fibrillation. N Engl J Med. 1975;29;259-62.

16. Pantridge JF, Adgey AAJ, Geddes JS, Webb SW. The Acute Coronary Attack. Tunbridge Wells, UK: Pitman Press; 1975. p131.
17. Mirowski M, Reid PR, Mower MM, Watkins L, Gott VL, Schauble JF, et al: Termination of malignant ventricular arrhythmias with an implanted automatic defibrillator in human beings. N Engl J Med. 1980;303:322-4.
18. Watkins L, Guarnieri T, Griffith LSC, Levine JH, Veltri EP, Juanteguy JM, et al: Implantation of the automatic implantable cardioverter defibrillator. J Cardiac Surg. 1988;3:1-7.
19. Kennedy DM. In search of Vivien Thomas. Tex Heart Inst J. 2005;32:477-88.
20. Kerber RE, Martins JB, Kienzle MG, Constatin L, Olshansky B, Martins B, et al. Energy, current, and success in defibrillation and cardioversion: clinical studies using an automated impedance-based method of energy adjustment. Circulation. 1988;77:1038-46.
21. Martens PR, Russell JK, Wolcke B et al. Optimal response to cardiac arrest study: defibrillation waveform effects. Resuscitation 2001;49:233-43.
22. Gliner BE, Jorgenson DB, Poole JE, White RD, Kanz KG, Lyster RD et al. Treatment of out-of-hospital cardiac arrest with a low-energy impedance-compensating biphasic waveform automatic external defibrillator. Biomed Instrum Technol. 1998;32:631-44.
23. Dalzell, GW, Cunningham, SR, Anderson J, Adgey AA. Electrode pad size, transthoracic impedance and success of external ventricular defibrillation. Am J Cardiol. 1989;64:741-4.
24. White NM, Parker WS, Binning RA, Kimber ER, Ead HW, Chamberlain DA. Mobile coronary care provided by ambulance personnel. BMJ. 1973;3:618-22.
25. Chamberlain DA, Vincent R, Mariba T, Saunders M. Historical vignette: the first cardiac first responders (letter). Resuscitation. 2014;85:e33-e34.
26. Baskett PJF. Use of Entonox in the ambulance service. BMJ. 1970;2:41-3
27. Baskett PJF, Diamond AW, Cochrane DF. Urban mobile resuscitation: training and service. Br J Anaesthesia. 1976;48:377-85.
28. Hyunh T, Birkhead J, Huber K, O'Loughlin J, Stenestrand U, Weston C et al. The prehospital fibrinolysis experience in Europe and North America and implications for wider dissemination. JACC Cardiovasc Interven. 2011;4:877-83.
29. Danne PD. Trauma management in Australia and the tyranny of distance. World J Surg. 2003;27:385-9.

30. Fedoruk JC, Paterson D, Hlynka M, Fung KY, Gobet M, Currie W et al. Rapid on-site defibrillation versus community program. Prehosp Disast Med. 2001;17:102-6.
31. O'Rourke MF, Donaldson E, and Geddes, JS. An airline cardiac arrest program. Circulation. 1997;96:2849-53.
32. O'Rourke RA. Saving lives in the sky. Circulation.1997;96:2775-7.
33. Brown AM, Rittenberger JC, Ammon CM, Harrington S, Guyette FX. In-flight automated external defibrillator use and consultation patterns. Prehosp Emerg Care. 2010;14:235-9.
34. Peterson DC, Martin-Gill C, Guyette FX, Tobias AZ, McCarthy CE, Harrington ST et al. Outcomes of medical emergencies on commercial airline flights. N Engl J Med. 2013;368: 2075-83.
35. Claesson A, Fredman D, Svensson L, Ringh M, Hollenberg J, Nordberg P et al. Unmanned aerial vehicles (drones) in out-of-hospital-cardiac-arrest. Scan J Trauma Resus Emerg Med. 2016;24:1-9.

Chapter 8

Evolution of Pre-Hospital Emergency Services

In medical circles and communities on both sides of the Atlantic, reports of early efforts to stem the tide of death from myocardial infarction or to reduce the carnage on the highways of an increasingly frenzied society were met often with apathy, sometimes with curiosity, and occasionally with excitement and the feeling that these medical dreamers were on to something.

We can say that the emergency medical services (EMS) system of today is the crop grown of the seeds sown by several hardy pioneers. They came from no single country, were of no one specialty, but they shared the necessary quality of the innovator - curiosity. And luck. Whatever forces, serendipity, or fate were at work when James Elam shared the car ride with Peter Safar in 1956 we can only be grateful, for out of that long-distance chat came the proof that expired air, delivered by mouth-to-mouth or mouth-to-nose, could maintain oxygenation.[1] Safar returned to Baltimore where, across town at Johns Hopkins Medical School and not far from his clinical and research base at Baltimore City Hospital, three eager scientists, Drs. Kouwenhoven, Knickerbocker and Jude, reported a fascinating chance observation as they were studying ventricular fibrillation and defibrillation in a dog. When the defibrillator paddles were placed firmly on the dog's chest, they noticed a - 'blip' - on the blood pressure tracing.[2] This seed sown by these basic and clinical scientists fell on some pretty fertile soil and grew fast. Within months of the 1960 paper from Johns Hopkins introducing the world to the technique of closed-chest cardiac massage,[3] (methods of ventilation, other than mouth-to-mouth were scarcely mentioned) Safar published his description of CPR - ventilation combined with closed-chest massage - and in which he also proved the failure of chest pressure alone to achieve adequate ventilation.[4] These techniques quickly spread around the world, so much so that an international symposium was convened in August 1961 in Stavanger, Norway, about three months after publication of the Safar paper. The recommendations of the assembled experts (the list of participants reads like an honour roll of pioneers in cardiopulmonary resuscitation) included enthusiastic acceptance of mouth-to-mouth/nose ventilation, closed-chest massage, widespread education of school children in these techniques, continued data collection and encouragement of ongoing research.[5]

Meanwhile, outside hospital

Before considering further the rapid progress towards eventual acceptance of these early observations and often serendipitous discoveries, it might be wise to reflect on what was, during the early part of the decade of the fifties, the current thinking, teaching and practice in the field of immediate care, emergency treatment or 'first aid.' We should pause and reflect on the fact that the medical sciences, and the research which drove them, were just beginning to see the results not only of scientific probing but also of more widespread and rapid dissemination of new findings. It took years for the methodical plodding of a Pasteur, a Lister, or a Nightingale to influence clinical surgery or hospital practice.[6]

Until the studies of Elam, Safar and their colleagues, little attention was paid by physicians to immediate care outside the operating theatre or the hospital. First aid was for Boy Scouts, life-saving societies, police or fire services or Red Cross volunteers - in other words the lay public. It was unusual for physicians or other health professionals to get involved in what appeared to be non-medical (i.e. non-physician) immediate care. Even paid ambulance drivers were considered to need very little, if any, training; many were volunteers, especially in Canada, the UK and Australia. High quality on-the-scene care in the event of accidents or sudden illness was provided, beginning in the late 19th century and even into the 21st, mostly by volunteer organisations such as the St. John Ambulance Society in countries connected with the British Empire, and the Red Cross world-wide.[7] However, in the American white paper on trauma, shock and anaesthesia of 1966, it was noted that 50% of civilian ambulance services were apparently owned and operated by morticians, most likely because they provided the only vehicle (hearses) in which the unfortunate citizen could recline, commonly alone and unattended, in the back of the vehicle.[8]

The research findings and subsequent action of James Elam and Peter Safar, boosted by the white paper, changed all that.[8] It is crucial to our story to note that Safar designed his original experiments in airway management and rescue breathing to demonstrate the clear superiority of mouth-to-mouth ventilation of non-breathing patients and used as subjects physicians, medical students and a nurse. Those performing the artificial respiration techniques, including both manual and expired-air breathing techniques, were Boy Scouts, firemen, and the Ladies Auxiliary

95

of the Baltimore City Hospital.[9] This study design remains as a testament to the vision and foresight of a dedicated, driven clinician-researcher who clearly saw these rescue techniques not as a procedure to be practiced only by physicians, or exclusively by health professionals, but as a relatively safe and effective method of saving lives in the hands of the general lay public.[10] Within months of the publication by Safar describing a technique of mouth-to-mouth ventilation combined with chest compression to provide life-sustaining blood flow,[4] the first international conference was convened in Stavanger, Norway to propose structured recommendations and add support to the widespread adoption of these techniques, emphasising the teaching of mouth-to-mouth breathing to all school children.[5]

During the decade of the fifties, and before the publication demonstrating the ability to sustain some circulation in the absence of effective heart action by chest compressions,[3] cardiac massage was performed through a chest incision and by directly squeezing the heart to produce forward blood flow. Success rates of this open-chest cardiac massage averaged 28% in a world-wide survey of 1200 patients reported in 1953,[11] prior to the work of Kouwenhoven and the Johns Hopkins Group.[3] It is important to note that almost all of the patients in this collection arrested in the operating theatre and had open-chest massage. This report has been occasionally cited as evidence that open-chest massage is superior to closed, but the comparison of apples inside the hospital and oranges outside the hospital is unhelpful. Up until the combined research reports and efforts of Kouwenhoven's[3] and Safar's[4] groups, many surgeons prepared themselves to open the chest for heart massage by carrying a scalpel in their wallets. In one case a fellow-surgeon awoke from a faint to find his *'colleague with a scalpel poised over his chest.'* [12] A rather veiled argument has been proposed for bringing back open-chest cardiac massage in non-trauma arrests,[13] despite there being no study comparing open and closed cardiac massage within the context of an EMS system, except for one post-trauma arrest report which demonstrated no higher survival rates in one method over the other.[14]

Although progress was being made in studying more effective ways of saving lives, particularly in the immediate management of airway problems or cardiac arrest, the major killer of younger people - accidental death - seemed to be accepted by most people as either inevitable, or the painful cost of the faster pace of life engendered by the automobile and industrial technology. There was a very practical reason for what appeared to be apathy, or at least a slow response to offer solutions to the growing problem. Quite simply, few knew how bad the problem was and, if they did know, there appeared to be no easy solution. All that changed in 1966 with the release of the now-famous white paper with the imposing and definitive title, *Accidental Death and Disability: the Neglected Disease of Modern Society*.[8]

Death, disability and the influence of war

The picture painted by this report, generated under the auspices of the National Academy of Sciences (NAS) through the National Research Council (NRC) of the United States,[15] painted a dismal picture of the state of accident and emergency services in that country.[8] Especially alarming was the chaos existing in what we now call pre-hospital care or emergency medical services. There was no system per se; ambulances varied in types, configuration, equipment, regulations required and personnel. Most ambulance drivers were negligibly trained, or not at all. There were no standards or requirements for education or training; ambulance vehicles were required only to have the capacity to carry a citizen reclining.[15] With 50% of ambulances owned and operated by morticians, personnel often did double-duty, serving as embalmers and funeral home assistants if not on a call. This chaotic state of affairs did not end at the hospital doors; frequently, those doors were locked, or if not the main entrance, the door to the emergency 'room' might be.

One of the main protagonists behind the 1966 report was Dr. John Howard, a former military surgeon who had served in the Korean conflict and has recently published an account of the influences which inspired the committee.[15] It is clear that the American experience in two conflicts - Korea and Vietnam - shaped the philosophy as well as the goals of the framers of this document. Their deliberations were influenced by military surgeons who had returned from these conflicts after having observed and participated in an efficient and effective system of trauma care which resulted, in both wars, in improved outcomes and the saving of lives.[16,17] Not only had military surgeons experienced an improved level of care for the seriously wounded on the battlefield,[18] but they had also trained medical corpsmen to perform life-saving interventions previously restricted to the domain of the physician.[17,19] What they saw in the non-system of civilian trauma care available to their families and fellow-citizens of the country they had defended, increased their dedication and determination that something better must be offered to the wounded on the highways and byways of America. Also increasing the pressure to improve civilian emergency care in America were the thousands of medics from the Korean theatre, and later paramedics from the Vietnam conflict. Many of these had, after demobilisation, entered the hospital system, public safety services (fire, police, fire rescue). Even those who became regular civilians never forgot the value they felt as military medics or, if not a medic, believed that those medics were there to save their lives.[19] So why not use them now, at home in America?

The report's unflinching - some would say scathing - verdict on the emergency care of illness and injury in modern American society rang true to many who read it. Among these were medical researchers, clinicians, interested citizens, benevolent community organisations, and progressive politicians who were becoming increasingly alarmed at the ragged quality of both emergency and primary care for a growing population and expanding middle class.[20]

Not that emergency care *inside* the hospital was necessarily any better, especially in the hidden areas which staff euphemistically called 'emergency rooms.' Staffing was a constant problem in the days and nights of the fifties and sixties, and in some places well beyond that. Junior house-staff, including first-year residents (then called 'Interns') who, perhaps a week before had been medical students, were expected to be in the forward trenches facing catastrophically injured patients, the seriously ill, and those in the process of dying.[21] Some hospitals' emergency rooms were staffed simply by a triage nurse who called a physician listed on the call rota.[22]

The NAS/NRC report was not the first voice crying amid the carnage. Earlier in the century the American College of Surgeons was actively lobbying for both a structured approach to the study and management of this major health problem and also for the immediate improvement in clinical care. Combining several other initiatives a Committee on Trauma was formed under the leadership of Dr. RH Kennedy, a vigorous critic, yet helpful promoter, of the state of emergency care in and out of the hospital.[23] Under his leadership the committee surveyed hospital administrations around the country and the results formed the basis for *A Guide to the Organization and Management of Hospital Emergency Departments*, reported by Kennedy in 1955.[24]

The dilemma faced by surgical organisations and by surgeons personally was that trauma care was not, in general, a popular field of practice for surgeons of the sixties. This was outlined in a 1961 editorial in the brand-new *Journal of Trauma* which rather starkly, and frankly, probed the reasons for this orphan but crucial field of care:

'Why is trauma care so unpopular? Either the injured patient intrudes on an already busy day or he demands care at night or on a weekend. He may or may not be an operative case and his convalescence may be prolonged. He does not come through the ordinary channels of referral but rather through assignment and while the patient may be grateful for his excellent care the surgeons will not therefrom build a practice. It would serve the surgeon better to treat, study and write in an elective field where his writings will attract patients from his colleagues.' [25]

It should be noted that no mention is made in this lamentation about the fact that most trauma patients, particularly in the fifties and sixties, were likely indigent, penniless and frequently charity cases, a not-inconsequential financial burden which the physician would be expected to bear. Although there were expressions of concern as to how to 'ensure excellent care for patients' surgeons and their official bodies presented few workable recommendations, and these usually focused on surgeons and their role, rather than taking a systems-approach to the growing problem. Plans, when they were presented at all, failed to address the weakest links in the chain - the 'emergency room' and ambulance care - and in at least one proclamation, dismissed both as irrelevant and recommended they be bypassed.[26] Not discussed was how the injured were to get to the hospital in the first place to receive care from the master surgeon mentioned in the editorial.[26]

The elements driving change were not limited to those in the harsh picture painted by the NAS/NRC committee. Viewing the situation from a broader perspective, the increased numbers of citizens swamping emergency rooms in the decades beginning with the fifties and continuing into the 21st century,* exposed the system to the scrutiny of the general public who eventually demanded improvements.[27] This pressure was felt by public officials, hospital administrators, clinicians and, eventually, organised medicine.

Efforts to address the problem began in earnest following the 1966 release of the NAS/NRC report and its dismal portrait of emergency care, both in and outside hospital. It had been previously recognised that a serious gap existed between in-hospital and outside-hospital emergency care. In fact, given the knowledge of the time, most physicians believed little could be done outside the hospital anyway.

---

* *From the 20th to the 21st century, in only 15 years, the total number of visits to emergency departments increased 34% (between 1995 and 2010 -from 97 million to 130 million visits) alone. Currently about 1 in 4 Americans visits an emergency department at least once a year*[27]

The usual mantra was, 'get-em-to-the-hospital-as-quick-as-you-can'; what happened in the interim, however brief, wasn't a priority. Visionary thinkers such as the surgeon RH Kennedy warned that *'...the improved forms of treatment are adopted by the medical profession, but may not be incorporated in first-aid books for years, because the professions did not know how to place them before a layman practically.'* [23] He worked hard to fill that gap by publishing, teaching and research, but it took time to alter the landscape.[28]

Several years before the critical report was issued, significant advances had been made in developing effective means of artificial respiration[29] and circulation,[3] and the term 'CPR' was introduced by both Dr. Safar[30] and, officially, by the American Heart Association in 1962.[31] Before that, in the late 1950's, Safar had begun to turn his attention to how this new CPR could be done outside the hospital, especially in a moving vehicle. Up to that time, few, if any ambulances in America could accommodate an attendant, even sitting.

Following their cooperation in the original airway studies using firemen as volunteer rescuers,[29] Baltimore Fire Chief Martin McMahon and Peter Safar had become close colleagues and friends, co-authoring one of the first papers to describe a mouth-to-airway modification of mouth-to-mouth ventilation.[32] McMahon became a crucial consultant in altering the design of an early ambulance to provide space for an attendant to perform CPR or ventilate the patient.[33] This was one of the first efforts to design a vehicle for patient transport and give priority to clinical care, especially resuscitation techniques. Submitted for publication over a year before the NAS/NRC report, this early paper was specific in its recommendations for equipment as well as referencing new standards for emergency attendants' training programmes. Meanwhile, in 1961, Peter Safar relocated to the University of Pittsburgh and already was working on a plan to develop a community approach to the provision of out-of-hospital emergency care which was, to him, a natural follow-up from his resuscitation research and his desire to train rescue workers in the technique. But his concept went well beyond the single, albeit important, aspect of airway control and ventilation. He envisioned the base of community out-of-hospital care to be resuscitation techniques by well-trained emergency attendants, but believed those personnel should have a much broader and structured training programme backed by ongoing research, and evidence-based protocols.

As the NAS/NRC was getting organised in the early 1960's, Safar was approached by one of the organisers from the National Research Council to join a subcommittee on community-wide Emergency Medical Services

(EMS), and later to serve as chairman of a subcommittee on ambulances.[34] Based on his continuing work in his new position as Professor and Chair of Anesthesiology at the University of Pittsburgh, Safar was able to promote his convictions nationally that emergency care workers needed training and standards, and an ambulance designed around the tasks the medics were called on to perform. As early as 1964 he documented what he felt was necessary for a community-wide emergency care system [35] and, in his position as chairman of the American Society of Anesthesiologists, he was able to influence the committee to propose national standards.[36] The bulk of these recommendations had previously been accepted internationally by the 2nd World Congress of the International Association for Traffic Medicine in Stockholm in September, 1966, the same month in which the NAS/NRC report was released.[37]

Safar and his group in Pittsburgh were not alone in their advocacy for better resuscitation efforts and emergency care in the streets. A newly-minted anaesthetist by the name of Eugene Nagel accepted a position at the University of Miami where, in1964 at Jackson Memorial Hospital, he met up with the equally-new Chief of Cardiovascular Surgery, Dr. James Jude, the same Jude of CPR fame who had been involved in research into defibrillation in Dr. Kouwenhoven's laboratory at Johns Hopkins.[3] Encouraged and inspired by Jude, Dr. Nagel took the lead and, beginning with the fire-rescue service in Miami, began diplomatically but persistently to advocate training of fire rescue personnel as paramedics. Nagel was convinced that the best and most efficient way to provide for emergency services in Miami was through the Fire Service which already had a system and telecommunications network in place to respond to calls for help from the public - almost any kind of help.[38] With what must be judged as the epitome of patience, forbearance and just plain grit, Nagel carefully, methodically and with due respect to all concerned crafted an approach which ultimately won most officials over. This included the demonstration of intravenous access and intubation skills by the paramedics, using himself as the subject.[39,40] (See Chapter 6)

It was the medical news from Belfast in 1967 (see Chapter 4) which spurred the ever-resilient Nagel towards his goal of increasing the role and responsibilities of the paramedic rescue units of the Fire Service and devising a training programme for them.[41] In the environment of the Fire Service and under the rather myopic scrutiny of its powerful Chief, Nagel began to build his case for extended training first by demonstrating that ventricular fibrillation was being met with by rescue units in the field and that by using space age technology, that is, telemetric transmission of the EKG signal and radio, the hospital-based physician could readily supervise care. Nagel was aware of the design of the Belfast model, which was based on a nurse-physician team aided by an ambulance attendant and occasional medical student. He however felt that the physician-led team approach would not be sustainable in the American system, at least not without major adjustments, and certainly not in the Miami system.[38] So he began by setting up a voice/radio and telemetry network as early as 1967 and reported on its progress at a medical conference in November of that same year.[42] Gradually, piece by piece, the Miami paramedic system began to take shape and a curriculum was developed. Nagel was one of the early EMS visionaries who taught and learned in solid partnership with the personnel in the system in a spirit of mutual respect, while depending on each other to mould the system to the needs of the community, both current and future. He envisioned, rather than a disease-specific service, a broader approach to emergencies within the community, and the system which he fostered evolved to what could better be described as an advanced life support emergency service.[38]

Telemetry allowed the transmission of an electrocardiographic signal from field units to a base hospital so that clinicians might advise field teams as to diagnosis and appropriate interventions. This technology became particularly attractive during the early years of EMS development because of the importance placed on cardiac rhythm disturbances, especially ventricular fibrillation, but it served as well to provide in-hospital physicians with at least a sense of indirect supervision of the field teams who were initiating care for their patients. In short, the use of telemetry offered a degree of security to physicians who invariably felt uncomfortable treating patients they could not see, hear or touch.[43] In his push to advance the paramedic rescue system in Miami-Dade area, Nagel considered telemetry to be useful in his step-by-step construction of the system as he sought to convince Fire administration of the value and safety of advanced pre-hospital care. His vision was that paramedics might be freed eventually from the telemetric leash as the technology faded out of use as both research and field experience demonstrated little benefit to it.[43,44] Newer technology was to replace it in the digital age.

The Pittsburgh renaissance

Even before *The Lancet* broke the news of the Belfast breakthrough[41] in America and around the world, precedent-setting developments were beginning to take shape not only in Eugene Nagel's Miami but also west of the Alleghenies, in the city of Pittsburgh. In that industrial city built along the banks of three rivers - the Monongahela and the Allegheny joining to form the Ohio - the city of Pittsburgh in the second half of the 20th century was busy cleaning up. Within several decades it would emerge from the soot and noon-hour darkness of smog into a colourful modern mix of cleaner skies, green spaces, rich ethnic mosaics, and centres known for academic excellence and technological ingenuity. In the decade of the sixties, the city was able to attract investment and leaders in the fields of commerce, government, research, medicine and health care. The University of Pittsburgh, surrounded on all sides with large teaching hospitals, was poised to foster centres of excellence in public health, ophthalmology, women's health, transplant surgery and other specialities, building largely on one of the most celebrated successes in modern public health – the Salk polio vaccine.[46]

Into this cauldron bubbling with ideas and promise a young, eager Peter Safar arrived from Baltimore as Chair of a new department, with the goal of cobbling together an academic programme in the growing specialty of anaesthesia using as a base the several university-affiliated hospitals carrying out up to 60,000 anaesthesia procedures yearly.[47] This father of CPR, as many have called him, had already shown his commitment to public health and his interest in ambulance services even in the basic research he designed to demonstrate the effectiveness of mouth-to-nose or mouth-to-mouth rescue breathing. It was Safar's vision that these techniques would be used by the lay public, and outside the confines of hospitals or clinics.[29]

Shortly after his arrival in Pittsburgh, Safar began to sketch out his concept of a community-based emergency medical services (EMS) programme. The ambulance service in the city of Pittsburgh in the early sixties was provided by the police and, as with other American towns and cities, offered only rudimentary assistance. As early as 1964 Safar had summarised standards for ambulance equipment and design, later updated for mobile intensive care and proposing that physicians must take leadership roles in improving first aid, ambulance transportation, and hospital emergency room coverage.[33,48] His initial principles, published in 1965, formed part of the ongoing discussions of the Committee on Acute Medicine of the American Society of Anesthesiologists which published their recommendations in 1968.[36]

Pittsburgh's unique 'make-work' project

Shortly before the arrival of Peter Safar, an energetic and idealistic young man arrived in Pittsburgh after education at Yale and work in Boston, to take up his position with The Hospital Planning Association in 1960.[49]

Phil Hallen's outlook and philosophy was unlikely to be lost in the reality of the poverty and despair so evident in some neighbourhoods in his adopted town. As an ambulance attendant during his earlier years, he had seen it all from the pavement up; yet he was struck by the racial divides and privation so evident in parts of the city, especially the district near the University Hospital known as 'The Hill.' With his medical experience, he was drawn to the sad state of Pittsburgh's ambulance service, largely assigned to the police and notable for being under-equipped and with attendants minimally trained, if at all. For Hallen the need for improvement was crystallised by the sudden cardiac death which struck down the former Governor of the State and mayor of the city, David Lawrence, during a political meeting in November, 1966, just two blocks from the University Hospital.[49] Distressed over the medical deficiencies in ambulance service evident in the management of the former Governor's sudden illness, Phil Hallen acted. Within months he drew up a plan for a not-for-profit ambulance service run by the newly-formed economic coalition '*Freedom House Enterprises Corporation*,' and staffed by trained attendants drawn from the ranks of the unemployed and, it was said, unemployable, young men of The Hill District.[50]

This initiative by Hallen was unique in several ways:

1. It was designed around the emergency medical needs of citizens as determined by those who knew what was lacking in the streets.
2. It was based on national standards which were developed only blocks down the hill from its headquarters at the University of Pittsburgh before these standards were even published by official medical organisations[49]
3. The curriculum was developed by physicians and others closely involved in resuscitation and other emergency procedures and was heavily slanted towards clinical skills backed by hands-on practice.
4. It provided an underserved and impoverished community with opportunities for education and social approval as well as gainful employment.[50]

In short, the organisation and curriculum could be justifiably known as 'Freedom House Paramedics,' and should be considered the first of the many systems which would be built on this national standard for paramedic education in the following decades.

It could be said of Freedom House that it was the first pre-hospital care system to have designated a street-level Medical Director responsible for education, standards, quality assurance and attending calls in the streets. Her name was Dr. Nancy Caroline, a member of the Critical Care Medicine programme under Peter Safar at the University of Pittsburgh. She quickly began to learn street medicine on-the-ground,[51] and won the admiration and loyalty of her paramedic students and colleagues, while enjoying the confidence of her mentor, Dr. Safar, and the Freedom House administration. In 1974 Safar delegated to Caroline the enormous task assigned to the University of Pittsburgh under contract from the US Department of Transportation: a review of training programmes and a survey of existing curricula in order to construct a national curriculum for training ambulance attendants.[34] Within two years she had succeeded in sorting through the myriad training programmes, role definitions, terminologies and testimonials, the expanse and challenge of her task expressed in an article she titled, *Would the real paramedic please stand up?* [52] (see also Chapter 9) Her findings and street-wise experience were later transformed into a text, *Emergency Care in the Streets*, which became the standard for lucid, coherent and comprehensible content relevant to the roles of a wide spectrum of emergency care providers.[53]

The impact of Belfast

As we have already seen (Chapters 3 and 4) Pantridge and Geddes fomented a revolution of sorts[54]- a bloodless one, more or less - but a revolution still. The spark that set them off was the startling fact that most people who succumbed to myocardial infarction did so within one to two hours of the onset of their symptoms.[55,56] Both clinicians had already suspected that their small coronary care unit - a few beds within the general medical ward at the Royal Victoria Hospital - was not having a dramatic effect on the death rate in the Belfast community and beyond. Worse perhaps was the feeling that even those who did get admitted were often in poor condition, and little could be done for them. Neither of the two cardiologists believed, at the time, that they were creating anything new or astounding; rather, they were applying logic to deal with the facts as they uncovered them - if most patients were dying before they could get to them, they would be obliged, in the immortal words of Clara Barton* during the American Civil War, to *'Treat them where they lie!'* [57]

---

* Clara Barton, was known as the "American Nightingale," and "The Angel of the Battlefield" who, although untrained, began early in the American Civil War to nurse the wounded often in the midst of battle. She later was instrumental in founding The American Red Cross.

And so they did. The whole idea of treating them where they lie was radical. Up to that time, on both sides of the Atlantic, ambulance services offered, at the most, a single service-transport of a citizen in a reclining position.[8] In many communities, there was only a driver, the patient was alone in the back, there was little if any room for an attendant anyway, and there were no standards or regulations.[33] The Belfast experiment went further; it brought the team and its technology to citizens in their homes, places of work, wherever they might be and treatment was initiated before transport was considered. It really was *treat them where they lie*. In addition, the pre-hospital interventions of the cardiac ambulance aimed to control the dysautonomia that often accompanied acute infarction, thus reducing the potential for the disaster of ventricular fibrillation. But it was suspected as well that the improvement of oxygenation, the management of pain and the treatment/prevention of arrhythmias would preserve myocardial tissue by maintaining coronary perfusion pressure and reducing ventricular workload.[58,59] It was not lost on the originators that the incidence of cardiogenic shock and pump failure fell noticeably in those patients treated beyond the walls of the hospital.[60] (See Chapter 5)

Cobbling together an elderly ambulance with a team of driver, nurse and physician, they broke radically from the convention that technologically-dependent treatments must be done in hospital and not anywhere else. This, in part, is what they set out to disprove, and in doing so they changed the practice of cardiology, as well as adding to the forward movement which had already begun elsewhere to improve the immediate treatment of the sick and injured. The timing of this revolution was, most would agree, fortuitous, occurring at the same time as a realisation was growing elsewhere, particularly in North America, that immediate care, whether offered in ambulances or emergency departments, was in an abysmal state.[8,21,22]

What Belfast was

The major achievement of the Pantridge and Geddes team was demonstrating that lives which ordinarily would have been lost could be saved. But the spinoff of their programme was the implicit challenge to any community to find a way to solve the problem of sudden cardiac death, and what was needed to solve it. Early on, a few communities and clinicians in both the UK and North America adopted the Belfast model. Most, however, opted to adapt to the circumstances in their communities, and soon were changing to a model which served the same ends but made use of those resources which were already in place outside the hospital. One or two jurisdictions, for reasons which we will examine, constructed a hybrid with significant involvement of physicians in the education programme and field work of their EMS systems.[61]

The improvement which the clinicians saw in overall death rates and the condition of patients who survived their initial acute ischaemic event reflected the role that time-to-treatment plays in the outcome of the disease. Belfast represents the beginning of a greater understanding of what many clinicians suspected - that intervening as early as possible to control autonomic dysfunction and to reduce ventricular workload could not only help prevent lethal arrhythmias, particularly ventricular fibrillation, but also might preserve myocardial tissue and reduce the incidence of resultant cardiogenic shock. [54,58,62] This latter 'pre-thrombolysis' supposition would become the focus of researchers and clinicians over the next several decades.[63,64] Thrombolysis, as eventually adopted in many pre-hospital systems, added to the potential for tissue salvage; a perhaps hoped-for, if not unintended, benefit of the Belfast approach. (See Chapter 5)

Sometimes lost in the celebration of the significance of the patients' outcome from the original paper is the fact that the Belfast cardiologists did not rest on their laurels. They continued to collect data, to share the details of their project with interested clinicians internationally, and to further analyse their results. Their analysis helped answer significant questions with respect to early management of acute ischaemic disease, one of which dealt with the energy levels required to defibrillate most patients in ventricular fibrillation.[65,66] This question was crucial, especially to pre-hospital services, since the larger the 'dose' delivered by a defibrillator, the larger and less portable the apparatus would have to be to deliver an effective shock. From early on in the project the Belfast team was hoping for a smaller, more compact defibrillator and had already put together a make-shift version which would later transform into the Pantridge Portable Defibrillator, weighing all of 3.2 kg.![67] This was heralded on the other side of the Atlantic by an article on the front page of the New York Times, with its proponent, Dr. Richard Crampton, (see Chapter 6) witness to the breakthrough that this Belfast contribution proved to be.[68] The article itself hinted at the potential for public access to defibrillators, coming close to the principle, if not exactly the device, we now know as automated defibrillation.

What Belfast was not

The daring medical experiment that was the cardiac ambulance in Belfast represented a trial of medical treatment by thoughtful clinicians outside the usual environment of the hospital and delivered as early as possible in the disease process. Two overriding elements were unique to the scheme - the environment and the earlier time of intervention. Pantridge and Geddes were acting logically on the fact that most patients suffering myocardial infarction died within minutes or hours of the onset of symptoms and therefore often beyond the reach of medical help. The system put in place sought to deliver a specialised team to the patient on receipt of a call from the family doctor and to assume the subsequent care. This system was not designed to answer calls for patients with chest pain or who suddenly collapsed. In the common parlance of the day, it was not a 'collapse- service.' Patients who were treated for ventricular fibrillation developed the complication either while the team was caring for them, or very shortly before the cardiac ambulance arrived on scene.[69]

Thus the 'Belfast model' was not designed to be a comprehensive emergency medical services system and never claimed to be one. Its patient base was filtered by the fact that general practitioners (GPs), educated to the system, made the call to the Pantridge team using a direct line to the coronary care unit, which depended entirely on the judgement of the house-call GP caring for the patient.[69] However, as the service developed, and its function and reputation clarified, direct calls from the public or from relatives of former patients might be directed to the CCU phone. This does not in any way diminish the revolution it caused or its world-wide effects, for the findings of their first report in *The Lancet* [41] were unprecedented and, as has been celebrated, a quite radical revolution.[54]

Lessons from Belfast

In short, the Belfast model was a specific, disease-focused experimental programme centred on the early management of acute myocardial infarction, with an emphasis on reducing the time-to-treatment, using a novel design - radical, perhaps - of taking treatment to citizens outside the confines of the hospital. It did not represent, nor was it designed to be, a full-service emergency medical system answering all calls to all people. But the spin-offs from this clinical trial were precedent-setting and long-lasting:

- Demonstrating the practicality of outside-hospital cardiac care, technology and all.
- Demonstrating the value of the early treatment of autonomic dysfunction secondary to ischaemia in preventing arrhythmias, particularly ventricular fibrillation.
- Early findings suggesting that time-to-treatment was crucial in

limiting myocardial damage, the time-is-tissue, tissue-is-time principle.

- Early proof that bigger isn't better- i.e. there was no need for any appreciable increase in the energy levels delivered by defibrillators with their increased risk of cardiac damage and post-shock arrhythmias.
- The development of a design and the manufacture of a light-weight defibrillator weighing less than 3.2 kg.

And finally, inspiring others to examine and freely adopt the lessons learned and the challenge to continue probing the science and the art of immediate, and at times life-saving, care.

The Belfast cardiologists shared data early in their project, welcomed visitors, continued to research and publish, and visited around the world to discuss their experience. The implications for ambulance services world-wide were far-reaching and the lessons from Belfast were central to the improvements slowly taking shape in pre-hospital emergency care on both sides of the Atlantic. It did not take long for those lessons to be transplanted to the pavements of New York and beyond.

Beyond Belfast

The impact of the 1967 *Lancet* article by Pantridge and Geddes announcing the results of their fifteen-month trial of mobile coronary care was quick to be felt, at least on the other side of the Atlantic. As outlined in chapter 6, mobile coronary care teams were assembled in New York (William Grace), Miami (Eugene Nagel), and Charlottesville, Virginia (Richard Crampton).[70-76]

Some elements of the Belfast model of mobile coronary care could not translate well to the American landscape. The methods, structure and practice of health care delivery in America was rapidly changing in the sixties (see Chapter 1), and even without those changes there remained significant differences when compared to the UK and continental Europe. As a result, the early disciples of Pantridge and Geddes had to make every effort to fit square pegs in round holes, and in most cases they came fairly close to being successful. It should be said that the American clinicians faced the same challenges as did their British counterparts in attempting to engender in their physician colleagues, hospital administrators and health system officials enthusiasm for their radical ideas. Pantridge himself remarked that health system officials, and even the Belfast media, at best were apathetic to the idea of mobile care, even after the publication of the 1967 paper.[60]

One of the systemic realities facing the American clinicians was the lack of an organised infrastructure for notification and communication. The Belfast model was purposely designed so that access to the system - i.e. activating the mobile team - was largely restricted to selected physicians who made house calls and they were considered an essential part of the project. They also had a standardised educational introduction to the system, which emphasised identification of ischaemic pain and other clinical findings which might trigger a call to the coronary care unit.[69] The several early programmes in America did not have a network of GP's who could triage patients and activate the mobile team if their clinical judgement required them to. Thus some programmes had to rely on lay dispatchers or public safety officers, who were medically untrained, to activate the mobile coronary care service. With the significant exceptions we have already noted, there seldom was an organised ambulance service within even urban areas, let alone in remote or rural communities. There existed *A patchwork of unregulated systems...with services sometimes being provided by hospitals, fire departments, volunteer groups or undertakers.'* [77] And rather than one hospital likely to be involved in one area, there were often several which might view with some alarm any system that appeared capable of diverting patients away from traditional referral patterns or of 'stealing' their patients.

Most challenging, however, was the fact that a physician member of the mobile team had to be supplied consistently and be hospital-based. This was difficult even in large teaching hospitals in which house staff had fixed assignments or rotations, and such staff were already in short supply. Even if resident physicians could be mobilised, there was no guarantee that a level of expertise in the area of coronary care could be achieved and maintained to a level appropriate to the sometimes complex needs of patients presenting with a wide spectrum of ischaemic cardiovascular disease.

However, the introduction of the Belfast system into the several urban teaching centres in the United States in the mid, and late sixties coincided with the in-depth examination of the quality of trauma care in the country by the National Academy of Sciences/National Research Council[8] This monumental report, excoriatingly critical in its tone and specifics, could not be ignored by government, media, or citizens. As a result, within a few years legislation was being prepared to fund Regional Medical Programs (RMP's) which sought to provide financial incentives to regions organised according to common needs and initiatives, not according to state lines or other formal jurisdictional boundaries.[78,79] These funds were distributed in the form of grants, therefore not committing the Federal Government to financially supporting programmes in perpetuity.[77] The funds for RMP's cut a wide swath, aimed at research and innovative clinical programmes involving heart disease, cancer and stroke. Because of the fact that immediate care could, broadly speaking, involve all three entities, emergency medical services became highly favoured when the distribution of funds came round. As a result, programmes for mobile coronary care benefited greatly; monies were allocated for training non-physician clinicians such as physician assistants, nurse practitioners and the newly-designated paramedics.

The infusion of cash into what had been, until the seventies, a neglected area of the health system - ambulance services - accelerated the improvement in EMS educational levels, curriculum development and mobile clinical care accelerated briskly across America.[77] The arrival of these funds promoted the change from physician/nurse-led teams for mobile coronary care (that term gradually evolving to mobile intensive care) to non-physician clinician teams (i.e. paramedics). These changes were further enhanced by private foundations, specifically the Robert Wood Johnson Foundation which announced its intention to fund forty-four EMS projects in an effort to force a more coherent approach to improving emergency services in the United States.[80] There was continued pressure by legislators and their physician allies to pass legislation providing programme funding for improving EMS systems. Testifying before the hearings on a proposed *EMS Development Act of 1973*, Peter Safar summed up the case for those pushing for the Bill: *'The state of EMS is...a disgrace, primarily because of lack of organization, coordination and clearly defined responsibilities and authorities....Implementation of national recommendations concerning ambulance services' improvement are still being retarded because of incompetence, bigotry, indifference of the public and governments, and because the interest of providers rather than consumers prevails.'* [81] Whether because of rhetoric, political manoeuvring or the justice of the cause, or all three, the *EHS Development Act of 1973* was passed only after the resignation of President Nixon and accession of Gerald Ford to the presidency.[82]

Spontaneous generation

Even before the passage of the EMS Act of 1973 and the funding which came from it, systems of pre-hospital care sprouted almost simultaneously in cities across America. Most addressed the toll of cardiovascular disease and were inspired by the Belfast experience. But each reflected the local available resources rather than being a mirror image of the Belfast structure. Few actually adopted the physician/nurse/ambulance attendant(s) construct, but all had one element in common in the beginning - strong physician leadership. Depending on the city or region, systems differed in regard to the composition of field teams, the extent of pre-hospital care that could be provided, the organisation providing the service and the training provided to field teams. Within several years of the 1967 *Lancet* paper from Belfast, systems of pre-hospital care were established in the UK, Europe and Australia, and almost all included physicians as part of the response teams. This was not the case in North America, due in part to the fact that emergency services were frequently provided by the fire services with ambulances provided by private companies, and so this model became the natural conduit for funding for any expanded role. The EMS Act of 1973 included a section on telecommunications and notification, including the adoption of a universal contact number, 911.[82]

By the time the EMS legislation was passed, EMS pilot programmes had been set up in at least six major American cities and, although highly influenced by the Belfast model, the favourable reports in the medical literature from the two Belfast-style programmes in the United States (Dr. Grace's programme in New York, Dr. Crampton's in Virginia) - served as American examples of meeting the needs of their local communities.[70,75,83] However, these two programmes were struggling to maintain the physician/ nurse element and remained focused only on the provision of out-of-hospital cardiac care. At least eight evolving programmes independently sprouted up across the United States in the period from the late sixties to the passage of the 1973 EMS Act:

- New York (Dr. Grace);
- Virginia (Dr. Crampton);
- Seattle (Dr. Cobb);
- Los Angeles (Drs, Criley/Lewis);
- Pittsburgh (Drs. Safar/Caroline);
- Portland, Oregon (Dr. Rose);
- Columbus, Ohio (Dr. Lewis);
- Long Island, Nassau County (Dr. Lambrew). (See Chapter 6)

It should be noted that the Belfast experience was known to, and influenced, these fledgling programmes and several of the physician leaders had visited Northern Ireland to see the Pantridge-Geddes set-up for themselves. Among the curious was a physician from the rural county of Haywood, North Carolina, a strikingly beautiful piece of America nestled in the Smoky Mountains. One of several local physicians had read the *Lancet* article describing the Belfast experience,[41] and decided to go see for himself. Dr. Ralph Feichter, an internist from the area, returned from Belfast intent on copying the main elements of the successful Belfast programme under a Regional Medical Program grant in 1968.[84] The key element to the success of this programme was the local volunteer Haywood County Rescue Squad, a high-quality, community-supported not-for-profit agency. Ambulance attendants were offered first aid training, progressing to higher levels of skills and responsibilities so that, within a year, *'The Haywood Rescue Squad entered history in 1969 as the first civilian, lay ambulance crews to perform invasive medical techniques.'* [85] This remarkable community-based service continues into the 21st century as an example of grass roots EMS, doing its job day-by-day, yet largely unsung.

Seattle takes the prize

When Leonard Cobb read the *Lancet* article by Pantridge and Geddes he thought it 'interesting,' and it was enough for him to realise he might have an ally in the Seattle Fire Department which already was providing emergency services to the public and First Aid training to its members.[86] He soon formed a partnership with a progressive Fire Chief, Gordon Vickery, who participated with Cobb in designing the 'tiered response' structure designed initially to get help to a stricken citizen as quickly as possible, at least to begin resuscitation techniques, with the second tier providing more advanced care. Cobb and Vickery agreed on the overall goals of the programme.[87]

1. To save lives of citizens;
2. To determine if non-physicians could manage CPR and carry out a cardiac arrest protocol;
3. To collect data, do research and to understand better sudden cardiac death.

They accomplished all three - and impressively so. The Medic I system was primed to go in 1970, and although physicians ran with the medic units for the first few months - mainly for education and supervision, not interventions - it was the intent of Cobb and Vickery to operate the system with paramedics managing the patients, with optional use of telemetry and radio contact with physicians at Harborview Hospital.

Seattle was unique in that the physician leadership formed a close partnership with a public entity, the Seattle Fire Service, and although the focus initially was on the management of sudden cardiac death, it provided a public health model of emergency care which ensured patient care/saving lives would remain as the guiding principle. The decision to expand the Medic I programme to include the citizens of Seattle as partners through the 'Citizen CPR' initiatives speaks to that guiding principle. The circle was complete; a public service agency (Fire), the medical element primarily from a teaching hospital (Harborview/University of Washington) and the citizens of King County. Running throughout this circle was a strong thread of research, the consortium contributing mightily to the medical literature and often leading the way with data that were crucial to shaping modern EMS systems in the United States and well beyond.

The Tinsel Town factor

The Los Angeles EMS paramedic programme predated the Seattle Fire-based project by a few months, but began as a medical research endeavour attempting to put in practice at least the principles of the Belfast model, if not the structure.[88] Three physicians, all cardiologists, led the way- Walter Graf, an influential member of the staff of a not-for-profit hospital near LAX airport, Michael Criley and James Lewis. Eventually they formed an alliance with the Los Angeles County Fire Department and the Los Angeles City Fire Department. Training programmes were set up at Daniel Freeman Hospital (Dr. Graf) and Harbor General Hospital, an affiliate of UCLA (Drs. Criley and Lewis).[89,90]

Although the system was set up to mirror the goals of the Belfast model, it was the intention of Criley and Lewis that fire rescue personnel (taking on the title 'paramedics' as in Seattle and Miami) would eventually operate without direct supervision of hospital-based nurses or physicians. Soon a legal conundrum raised its predictable, but ugly, head. At the beginning of the pilot programme, non-physician clinicians, except for CCU and ICU nurses, could not perform what were then defined under the law of California as 'medical acts.' These were limited to licenced physicians and would have included defibrillation, IV placement, intubation and the administration of drugs - particularly narcotics. When the programme started, rather than delay any longer, the paramedic unit first picked up the CCU nurse from Harbor General hospital and sped to the scene, following the initial response by another rescue truck or, more likely, a fire engine. This obviously occasioned delay in providing advanced care at the scene; the situation needed a solution - and fast. The Harbor General group found an ally in a local County Supervisor, Mr. Kenneth Hahn, who took the issue to the State legislators and eventually to Governor Ronald Regan. The result was the Wedworth-Townsend Paramedic Act passed in 1970 and amended in 1971.[91] Problem solved.

Figuring largely in the rapid expansion of the LA programme was the fact that an unlikely ally in the form of a Hollywood executive producer, Robert Cinader, whose passion for the Fire Service and all it represented was exceeded only by his creative genius. Cinader, under the watchful eye of his domineering mentor Jack Webb, saw in this new paramedic programme a different kind of medical drama - one that would involve going *outside* the hallowed walls of the hospital. He quickly grasped the elements of the LA programme, immersing himself, as did his writers, in the fire service and its culture surrounding the new paramedics. The result was the world premiere of a TV series which would run for years, and in syndication is still running, world-wide. *Emergency!* made its debut in January, 1972. The influence of this show is widely recognised not only on the careers of future physicians and EMS personnel, but also on legislative and legal debates and proceedings in the United States and perhaps globally.[91,92]

Pittsburgh's hybrid

The foundation for advanced pre-hospital care, as we have seen already, was laid down in the late sixties by dedicated leaders in the Pittsburgh community including Phil Hallen, Peter Safar and the Board of Freedom House Enterprises, an economic and social development agency based in the heart of the city, the Hill District.[49] Despite the growing evidence that Freedom House Ambulance was developing as a mature and valuable addition to health care in the city, by 1975 the service was shut down, having been starved of funds, and was withering beneath the darkening shade of acrimonious debate between the Mayor and Dr. Safar.[93] By 1978 after a new mayor was sworn in, the City of Pittsburgh Division of EMS was formed, but it was built on the concrete foundations of the Hill District.

The late 1970s saw a renaissance develop in Pittsburgh which clearly arose out of the previous Freedom House programme. Dr. Safar had worked to bring in a medical director whose emergency medicine and emergency medical services training fitted him for the task of rebuilding, while he then turned his considerable energy to resuscitation research while available for consultation and support for the new director. The new Medical Director of the Division of EMS (Dr. Ronald Stewart, a Canadian physician who trained as one of the first emergency medicine residents in the Los Angeles programme) was also the Director of the University Hospital Emergency Department and an active Associate Professor in the Pittsburgh School of Medicine. While attempting to learn as much as possible about the training and capabilities of the paramedics of the city, the Medical Director was thrust into the public spotlight when an iron worker atop one of the city bridges became trapped and required an on-scene disarticulation of the right knee some forty metres above the Monongahela River.[94] The event created such positive publicity for the paramedics of that city that the plans for a real renaissance of EMS and the further expansion of emergency medicine as a specialty were accelerated, and probably made easier, in large measure as the result of the tragedy of a patient losing a limb.[94,95]

The plan for the emergency medicine programme in Pittsburgh was greatly enhanced by the previous work done by Safar and Caroline, and the trail-blazing done by the Freedom House personnel and organisation. Necessary to any progress was the gradual but close liaison which developed with the EMS Division of the City. Within six months of the arrival of Stewart, the Centre for Emergency Medicine was formed and supported by a consortium composed of the University and teaching hospitals in the city.[95,96] A residency soon followed in 1981, a crucial component of which was the requirement for residents to be trained in EMS - in the streets, in the tradition set down by Nancy Caroline a decade earlier. [61,96] The influence of the Belfast group and the European model was evident in this Pittsburgh hybrid system which relied on paramedic practitioners partnered with physicians, both physician faculty from the Department of Emergency Medicine at the University and their residents. Belfast might even have been proud.

The movement down under

The lessons of Belfast were soon being learned around the globe, not the least or last of which were in Australia. That country faced challenges similar to those of Canada and the United States - compact urban populations surrounded by vast stretches of rural spaces, all in turn surrounded by oceans. Australia had a sound organisational tradition of ambulance services dating from the late nineteenth and early twentieth centuries which made easier the transition from a basic 'first-aid service' to more comprehensive pre-hospital care systems. The formation of St. John Ambulance corps throughout the Australian Commonwealth began during the early years and persist today, either to provide 'first aid' and humanitarian services to the population or, in Western Australia (WA) and Northern Territory (NT), is contracted by the government to provide emergency and transport services. In all other states emergency medical services are provided by State government as a third-service public agency.

Building on the foundations of the already-existing ambulances services in the states and territories, physician and community leaders became quickly aware of the Belfast experiment in late 1967, only a few months after its publication.[41] For several years following there began to build a movement to augment the in-place ambulance services with additional educational programmes, most notably in Sydney in the early seventies out of St. Vincent's Hospital,[97] and as well from Melbourne around the same time.[98] In the mid-seventies Dr. Bob Wright of St. Vincent's visited the Los Angeles programme, headed at the time by a Canadian, Ron Stewart. The structure of the Los Angeles fire service-based system in Los Angeles County appeared inappropriate for the Australian model of ambulance service, but the educational programme used evoked a major interest in Dr. Wright. Return visits by Stewart to Sydney, Melbourne and to fledgling paramedic programmes in the rest of Australia over the next ten years forged a solid bond across the Pacific.[99]

The decades since have seen Australia leading the way in educational research and curriculum development, with Dr. Frank Archer, now a Professor Emeritus of Monash University, internationally recognised for his work. Throughout the university systems in Australia there has been significant work done in the justification for and design of degree programmes to meet the need of the growing paramedic profession, especially in the field of basic and clinical research.

To meet the challenges of 'the tyranny of distance' in the vast country regions as well as the inner urban centres, regional trauma systems have been put in place and reported for the benefit of an eager global audience.[100] In respect to pre-hospital coronary care, EMS physicians and paramedics continue to report on their experience from the closely-monitored clinical pre-hospital practice environment, which has always been the hallmark of Australian emergency medical service systems

Building a subspecialty

At the national level in the United States, the creation of the *American College of Emergency Physicians* in 1968 and in the UK advocacy groups such as the *British Association of Immediate Care Schemes (BASICS)* in 1977, supported the sections of the Royal Colleges in both Britain and Canada as there began a movement towards the development of the new specialty. (see Chapter 9).

EMS personnel nationally were represented in America by the *National Association of EMTs* (Emergency Medical Technicians), founded in 1975, although other agencies and non-governmental agencies, such as the Red Cross, Heart and Stroke Associations, Trauma Societies, etc. shared common goals with these emergency care entities.

The evolution of EMS programmes continued in several directions, influenced by national initiatives designed to represent the interests of practitioners and projects around the United States which depended, initially at least, on Regional Medical Program (RMP) funding. The transition to permanent funding was not easy, and depended largely on the success of various programmes within communities. A key element was the continued visibility and advocacy of physicians active in the systems, a stated goal of the *National Association of EMS Physicians*[102] as well as *The American College of Emergency Physicians*.

Early efforts were evident in the field of communication and publishing. *Paramedics International*, a magazine originating in Los Angeles and its paramedic system in 1976, and which reflected street medicine in living colour. It later was purchased by James O. Page, a former Fire Chief with the Los Angeles County Fire Department. Jim Page became an EMS legend, building the magazine up to become one of the most widely-read publications in the early days, and beyond of EMS. His contributions were legion, as a lawyer and then CEO of the *Acute Coronary Treatment (ACT) Foundation,* he wrote legislation in many states and several countries and was a scholar and a leader in the field until his tragic and unexpected death in 2004.[103] His early publication efforts have been expanded and given rise to *JEMS: The Journal of Emergency Medical Services* which hosts some of the largest conferences, *EMS Today*, both of which cater to emergency personnel the world over and are now a subsidiary of Pennwell Corporation (USA).

Nothing new under the sun

Often overlooked in the evolution of out-of-hospital emergency medical services is the role of the Obstetric 'Flying Squad' in mid 20th century Britain. This was originally suggested in 1929 by Farquhar Murray, Professor of Midwifery and Gynaecology at the University of Durham.[104] In Britain, at that time, most maternity patients were managed at home by midwives and general practitioners (GPs). A major cause of maternal death was obstetric haemorrhage, and Murray suggested: '.....*instead of rushing a shocked and collapsed patient to hospital for nursing and specialised aid, the specialist and nurse should be rushed to the patient.*' [104,105] In 1931, the first fully organised flying squad service was run from Bellshill Maternity Hospital in Scotland.[106] The ambulance was staffed by an obstetrician, a midwife

118

and, sometimes, an anaesthetist. The aim was to provide back-up to the domiciliary midwife and GP, and help manage obstetric complications on site, followed by transportation of the mother and baby to the hospital as needed. Early anaesthetic equipment consisted of a Schimmelbusch mask and chloroform – some units later used more elaborate equipment and drugs.[107] Intravenous fluids and blood transfusion became important components – as well as drugs to control eclampsia.

During the 1930s to 1960s obstetric flying squads were established in most areas of the UK, particularly in the cities.[108] Although it was mainly a UK entity, the obstetric flying squad was also set up in response to local needs in other countries.[109,110] By the 1980s, a combination of fewer home births and the increased efficiency and resuscitation-capability of the general ambulance service, led to the discontinuation of most obstetric flying squads.[111] It might well have been considered the harbinger of things to come.

When all is said and done

It can convincingly be argued that the bold Belfast Experiment was the genie let out of the pre-hospital care bottle, not only because of the structural change in clinical care delivery it engendered - a medical flying squad - but rather because it represented a radical change from the traditional hospital-focused specialty care.[62] The success of Belfast and the logic of its philosophy - the sooner one treats, the better - was quickly realised internationally once The Lancet article[41] was released to the world. As we have already noted, coincident with the news from Pantridge and Geddes, gathering across the Atlantic were forces which were to play a major role not only in the configuration and structure of emergency care systems but also in the legislation and funding necessary to their development. The merging of these two revolutionary elements - mobile coronary care and the crusade to conquer the chaos and needless deaths on highways, in factories and in the homes of America and beyond - produced the impetus which triggered the evolution that shaped what became a crucial underpinning of our health system- emergency medical services.

References

1. Safar P. Careers in anesthesiology: an autobiographical memoir. Park Ridge, IL: Wood Library-Museum of Anesthesiology; 2000. p 129-30.
2. Eisenberg MS. Life in the Balance: emergency medicine and the quest to reverse sudden death. New York: Oxford University Press; 1997. p 122.
3. Kouwenhoven WB, Jude JR, Knickerbocker GG. Closed-chest cardiac massage. JAMA1960;1064-67.
4. Safar P, Brown TC, Holtey WJ, Wilder RJ. Ventilation and circulation with closed-chest cardiac massage in man. JAMA 1961; 176:574-6.
5. Stavanger Symposium. Recommendations of the symposium on emergency resuscitation. JAMA 1961;178:48.
6. Larson E. Innovations in health care: antisepsis as a case study. Am J Public Health 1989;79:92-9.
7. Bell RC. The Ambulance: a History. Jefferson, NC: McFarland & Company; 2009. p 126-36.
8. Committee on Trauma, Shock and Anesthesia. Accidental Death and Disability: the Neglected Disease of Modern Society. Washington DC: National Academy of Sciences-National Research Council; Sept,1966.
9. Safar P. Careers in anesthesiology: an autobiographical memoir. Park Ridge, IL: Wood Library-Museum of Anesthesiology; 2000. p 133-4.
10. Milka M. Peter J. Safar, MD: "Father of CPR," innovator, teacher, humanist. JAMA 2003; 289:2485-6.
11. Stephenson HE, Reid LC, Hinton JW. Some common denominators in 1200 cases of cardiac arrest. Ann Surg 1953; 137:731-44.
12. Julian DG: The evolution of the coronary care unit. Cardiovasc Res. 2001;51:621-4.
13. Kornhall DK, Dolven T. Resuscitative thoracotomies and open chest cardiac compressions in non-traumatic cardiac arrest. World J Emerg Surg 2014;9:54.
14. Bradley MJ, Bonds BW, Chang L, Yang S, Hu P, Li H, et al. Open chest cardiac massage offers no benefit over closed chest compressions in patients with traumatic cardiac arrest. J Trauma Acute Care Surg 2016;81:849-54.
15. Howard JM. Historical background to Accidental Death and Disability: the Neglected Disease of Modern Society. Prehospital Emerg Care 2000; 4:285-89.
16. Haacker MC. Time and its effects on casualties in World War II and Vietnam. Arch Surg 1969; 98:39-40.

17. Neel S. Army aeromedical evacuation procedures in Vietnam: implications for rural America. JAMA 1968;204:99-103.
18. Meier DR, Samper ER. Evolution of civil aeromedical helicopter aviation. Southern Med J 1989 ;82:885-91.
19. De Lorenzo RA, Lairet JR, Mothershead JL. Military Systems. In: Cone DC, O'Connor R, Fowler R, editors. Emergency Medical Services: Clinical Practice and Systems Oversight. Kendall/Hunt Publishing: Dubuque, IA; 2009. p 308-18.
20. Merritt AK. The rise of emergency medicine in the sixties: paving a new entrance to the house of medicine. J Hist Med Allied Sci 2014; 69:251.
21. Zink BJ. Anyone, Anything, Anytime: a History of Emergency Medicine. Philadelphia: Mosby; 2006. p 14-16.
22. Ibid, p 13.
23. Kennedy RH. Our fashionable killer: oration on trauma. Bull Am Coll Surg 1955;40:73-82.
24. Kennedy RH. Raising standards of care in the emergency department. Hospitals 1962;36:74-85.
25. Cassebaum WH. Does the injured patient receive optimal care? (editorial) J Trauma 1961;1:442-3.
26. Avellone JC. Emergency services for the severely injured. (editorial) J Trauma 1965;5:436-7
27. National Center for Health Statistics. Health, United States, 2012: Special Feature on Emergency Care. Hyattsville, MD. 2013. p 20.
28. Kennedy RH. Presidential address: problem areas in the surgery of trauma. Am J Surg 1956;91:457-60.
29. Safar P, Escarraga LA, Elam JO. A comparison of the mouth-to-mouth and mouth-to-airway methods of artificial respiration with chest-pressure arm-life methods. N Engl J Med 1958; 258:671-77.
30. Safar P. Careers in anesthesiology: an autobiographical memoir. Park Ridge, IL: Wood Library-Museum of Anesthesiology; 2000. p 144-5.
31. Eisenberg MS. Life in the Balance: emergency medicine and the quest to reverse sudden death. New York: Oxford University Press; 1997. p 132.
32. Safar P, McMahon M. Mouth-to-airway emergency artificial respiration. JAMA 1958; 166:1459-60.
33. Safar P, Brose RA. Ambulance design and equipment for resuscitation. Arch Surg 1965; 90:343-8.
34. Safar PJ. On the history of emergency medical services. Bull Anesth Hist 2001;19;1-11.
35. Safar P. Community-wide cardiopulmonary resuscitation. J Iowa

Med Soc 1964;11:629-35.

36. Committee on Acute Medicine American Society of Anesthesiologists. Community-wide emergency medical services. JAMA 1968; 204:133-40.

37. Safar P. Community-wide emergency care for acutely life-threatening conditions. Proc. 2nd Congress of International Association for Accident and Traffic Medicine, September 1966, Stockholm, Sweden: Skanetryck Publications;Malmo, Sweden.

38. Nagel E. History of emergency medicine: a memoir. Bull Anesth Hist 2001;19:1,9-10.

39. Eisenberg MS. Life in the Balance: emergency medicine and the quest to reverse sudden death. New York: Oxford University Press; 1997. p 227-8.

40. Ibid, p 231.

41. Pantridge JF, Geddes JS. A mobile intensive-care unit in the management of myocardial infarction. Lancet 1967;1:271-3.

42. Nagel EL, Hirschman JC, Mayer PW, Dennis F. Telemetry of physiological data: an aid to fire-rescue personnel in a metropolitan area. Southern Med J 1968;61:598-601.

43. Stewart RD. When less is more: Teflon and telemetry in the space age. (editorial) Ann Emerg Med 1985;41:992-4.

44. Pozen MW, Fried DD, Voigt GG. Studies of ambulance patients with ischemic heart disease. II. Selection of patients for ambulance telemetry. Am J Pub Health 1977;67:532-5.

45. Safar P. Careers in anesthesiology: an autobiographical memoir. Park Ridge, IL: Wood Library-Museum of Anesthesiology; 2000. p 206-7.

46. Laurence WL. Salk polio vaccine proves success; millions will be immunized soon; city schools begin shots April 25. New York Times.1955 Apr 13: p 1 (col. 8).

47. Safar P. Careers in anesthesiology: an autobiographical memoir. Park Ridge, IL: Wood Library-Museum of Anesthesiology; 2000. p 164.

48. Safar P, Esposito G, Benson DM. Ambulance design and equipment for mobile intensive care. Arch Surg 1971;102:163-71.

49. Bell RC. The Ambulance: a History. Jefferson, NC: McFarland & Company; 2009. p 256-76.

50. Benson DM, Esposito G, Dirsch J, Whitney R, Safar P. Mobile intensive care by "unemployable" blacks trained as emergency medical technicians (EMT's) in 1967-69. J Trauma 1972;12:408-21.

51. Caroline NL. Medical care in the streets. JAMA. 1977;237:43-6.

52. Caroline NL. Will the real paramedic please stand up? Emerg Med Services 1977;6:16-18,85.

53. Bedsoe B, Sanders MJ. A tribute to Nancy Caroline, MD, and Emergency Care in the Streets. JEMS 2002; p 127-9.
54. Eisenberg MS, Pantridge JF, Cobb LA, Geddes JS. The revolution and evolution of prehospital cardiac care. Arch Intern Med 1996;156:1611-19.
55. Yater WM, Traum AH, Brown WG, Fitzgerald RP, Geisler MA, Wilcox BB. Coronary artery disease in men eighteen to thirty-nine years of age. Am Heart J 1948;36:481-526.
56. Bainton CR, Peterson DR. Deaths from coronary heart disease in persons fifty years of age and younger. N Engl J Med 1963;268:569-75.
57. Metzger JC, Marcozzi DE. Tactical EMS. In: Cittone GR, editor. Disaster Medicine. 1st ed. Philadelphia: Mosby; 2006. p 297.
58. Pantridge JF. The effect of early therapy on the hospital mortality from acute myocardial infarction. (abstract) Quart J Med 1970;39:621-2.
59. Crampton RS. Frank's legacy from a North American perspective. Ulster Med J 2010;79(suppl 1):4-9.
60. Pantridge JF, Wilson C. A history of prehospital coronary care. Ulster Med J 1996; 65:68-73.
61. Stewart RD, Paris PM, Heller MB. Design of a resident in-field experience for an emergency medicine residency curriculum. (abstract) Ann Emerg Med 1985;14:491.
62. Pantridge JF. Mobile coronary care. Chest 1970;58:229-34.
63. Appleby P, Baigent C, Collins R, Flather M, Parish S, Peto R. Indications for fibrinolytic therapy in suspected acute myocardial infarction: collaborative overview or early mortality and major morbidity results from all randomised trials of more than 1000 patients. Lancet 1994; 343:311-22.
64. Welsh RC, Travers A, Senaratne M, Williams R, Armstrong PW. Feasibility and applicability of paramedic-based prehospital fibrinolysis in a large North American center. Am Heart J 2006;152:1007-14.
65. Pantridge JF, Adgey AAJ, Geddes JS, Webb SW. The Acute Coronary Attack. Tunbridge Wells: Pitman Medical; 1975. p 67-71.
66. Gascho JA, Crampton RS, Cherwek ML, Sipes JN, Hunter FP, O'Brien WM. Determinants of ventricular defibrillation in adults. Circulation 1979;60:231-40.
67. Baskett P. Frank Pantridge and the world's first miniature portable defibrillator. Resuscitation. 2005;65:5.
68. Altman LK. Portable heart unit is developed. New York Times. 19745 Aug 11; p. 1 (col.2-4).
69. Pantridge JF, Adgey AAJ, Geddes JS, Webb SW. The Acute Coronary

Attack. Tunbridge Wells:Pitman Medical; 1975. p 7.

70. Grace WJ, Chadbourn JA. The mobile coronary care unit. Dis Chest 1969;55:452-5.

71. Bell RC. The Ambulance: a History. Jefferson, NC: McFarland & Company; 2009. p288.

72. Dr. William J. Grace of St. Vincent's dies: was first head of a US hospital to use mobile emergency unit for victims of heart attack. New York Times. 1977 Feb 19;Sect. OB:26 (col.1-2).

73. Pantridge JF, Geddes JS. Cardiac arrest after myocardial infarction. Lancet 1966;i:807-8.

74. Eisenberg MS. Life in the Balance: emergency medicine and the quest to reverse sudden death. New York: Oxford University Press; 1997. p 221-2.

75. Crampton RS, StillermanR, Gascho JA. Prehospital coronary care in Charlottesville and Albemarle County. Virginia Med Mon 1972;99:1191.

76. Bell RC. The Ambulance: a History. Jefferson, NC: McFarland & Company; 2009. p 279-80.

77. Shah MN. The formation of emergency medical services system. Am J Public Health 2006; 96:414-23.

78. Chambliss CR. Regional medical programs: a new model for health care. J Natl Med Assoc 1969;61:25-30.

79. Wilbur DL. Quality and availability of health care under regional medical programs. JAMA 1968;203:945-9.

80. Request for proposals. National competitive program of grants for regional emergency medical communications systems. Princeton, NJ: Robert Wood Johnson Foundation; 1973.

81. Emergency Medical Services Systems Development Act of 1973. Hearings 93rd Congress. 1st Session., on 504 and 654. Washington, DC. United States Congress. Senate Committee on Labor and Public Welfare. Subcommittee on Health; 1973.

82. Emergency Medical Services Systems Act of 1973. (PL 93-154). Legislative History. Washington, DC; 1973.

83. Crampton RA, Aldrich RF, Gascho JA, Miles JR, Stillerman R. Reduction of prehospital, ambulance and community coronary death rates by the community-wide emergency cardiac care system. Am J Med 1975;58:151-185.

84. Bell RC. The Ambulance: a History. Jefferson, NC: McFarland & Company; 2009. p 278-84.

85. Ibid, p 282.

86. Eisenberg MS. Life in the Balance: emergency medicine and the

quest to reverse sudden death. New York: Oxford University Press; 1997. p233.

87. Ibid, p 234.

88. Lewis AJ, Ailshie G, Criley JM: Pre-hospital cardiac care in a paramedical mobile intensive care unit. Calif Med 1972;117:1-8.

89. Graf WS, Solin SS, Paegel BL. A community program for emergency cardiac care. A three-year coronary ambulance/paramedic evaluation. JAMA 1973;226:156-60.

90. Lewis AJ, Criley JM. (editorial) An integrated approach to acute coronary care. Circulation 1974;50:203-5.

91. Bergman P. Emergency! Send a TV show to rescue paramedic services. University of Baltimore Law Review 2007;36:347-69.

92. Yokley R, Sutherland R. Emergency! Behind the scene. Sudbury, MA: Jones and Bartlett; 2008.

93. Bell RC. The Ambulance: a History. Jefferson, NC: McFarland & Company; 2009. p 275.

94. Stewart RD, Young JC, Kenney DA, Hirschberg JM. Field surgical intervention: an unusual case. J Trauma 1979;19:780-3.

95. Zink BJ. Anyone, Anything, Anytime: a History of Emergency Medicine. Philadelphia: Mosby; 2006. p 203.

96. Gigler R. Pittsburgh Press. Emergencies are their specialties. 1981 Dec 13; p 4-5.

97. O'Rourke M. Modified coronary ambulances. Med J Austral. 1972 Apr;1:875-878.

98. Luxton MP, Thomas P, Richard H et al. Establishment of the Melbourne mobile intensive care service. Med J Austral. 1975 May;1:612-615.

99. Wright R, O'Rourke M. St Vincent's Hospital Sydney and the development of the NSW Ambulance Service. St Vincent's Clinic Proc. 2015;23:3-5.

100. Danne PD. Trauma management in Australia and the tyranny of distance. World J Surg. 2003;27:385-9.

101. Johnson S, Brightwell R, Ziman M. Paramedics and pre-hospital management of acute myocardial infarction: diagnosis and reperfusion. Emerg Med J. 2006;23:331-4.

102. Cone, DC, Brice JH, Delbridge TR, Myers, JB. (eds) Emergency Medical Services: Clinical Practice and Systems Oversight, Second Edition, John Wiley & Sons, Ltd: Chichester,UK;2015.

103. Bayot J. James Page, 68, advocate of emergency services dies. New York Times. Sept 21, 2004.

104. Murray EF. The organisation of a maternity service. BMJ. 1929;1:691.

105. Murray EF. The obstetrical "Flying Squad." BMJ. 1938;1:654-6.

106.Liang DY. The emergency obstetric service, Bellshill Maternity Hospital. J Obstet Gynaecol Br Cwlth 1963;70:83-93.

107.Davies CK. Anaesthesia for an obstetric flying squad, Br J Anaesth 1969;41:545-50.

108.Discussion on Emergency Obstetrical Services (The Flying Squad); its use and abuse. Proc Roy Soc Med 1949; 42:1-10.

109.Hagberg CJ. The Cape Town Obstetric Flying Squad: its inception, organization and operation. South Afr Med J 1956;30:1140-44.

110.Menon R. Experience of a rural obstetric flying squad service. Med J Malaya 1971;41:30-3.

111.Chamberlain G, Pearce JM. The Flying Squad. BJOG 1991; 98:1067-69.

Chapter 9

Development of the specialty of Emergency Medicine

From the 1950s onward, and for reasons already outlined, emergency rooms were fast changing to become the point of contact not only for increasingly important hospital services but also for access to primary and critical care. In the United States, it was widely reported in the health literature that emergency room visits were climbing at an alarming rate in the decade up to 1964, increasing by sixteen million (175%).[1,2]

Such increases rang alarm bells amongst hospital administrators and even some physicians, one of whom warned physicians to *'think through the serious social implications of this phenomenon and the part we unwittingly play in the momentum toward institutional medicine.'*[2] While such thinking might be akin to the crew of the Titanic wishing the iceberg would move out of the way, there appeared to be no consensus among organised medical groups or health care administrators as to what could be done with the emergency room problem. Not only were the number of visits increasing at an unprecedented rate throughout the sixties, this situation has continued into the 21st century so that at the end of the first decade of the new century, one in four Americans make use of emergency departments at least once a year, for a total of 130 million visits.[3] The dilemma facing hospitals was, and still is, not confined to the *number* of citizens crowding the hallways and stretchers of their emergency departments, but the *types* of patients who were being seen there. As the numbers increased, the spotlight was trained on *who* was there and *why* they were there. It was quickly realised that more than two-thirds of patients seen in the *'emergency room'* could not, in retrospect, be considered to constitute emergencies at all.[2] Most, in the opinion of several practitioners writing in the sixties, could be readily handled by private offices or clinics. The debate around what constitutes an emergency continued to rage, the strongest opinions coming from practitioners who may only have heard about, rather than suffered, a thrombosed haemorrhoid at midnight. Grave warnings about the volume of patients began to appear in the literature, some being incisively accurate:[2]

'If this trend continues and patients more and more seek the non-personal physician to handle his medical problems, it will not be too long before we will be faced with institutional medicine, not because the government is foisting it upon the people but because people are seeking medical care away from the family doctor.'

More accurately stated perhaps, the citizens were foisting this major change on the health care system and practitioners. Not surprisingly, most discussions of this problem eventually mentioned the issues of cost and fee structures. Examined superficially, it could be argued that patients were coming to emergency rooms because they were unable to access health care elsewhere. One obvious way to cure the problem was to offer primary care at another venue; perhaps a *'health clinic'* preferably with fewer bits of diagnostic technology, using a variety of practitioners, and therefore costing less. However, when closely examined, it was found that patients, even though registered in community health centres, continued to use the emergency department of large hospitals as a source of primary care *even when the community centre was open*.[4] Other practitioners, particularly those whose primary interest was in major trauma, understandably dismissed the emergency room of the era as irrelevant to trauma care and insisted it be bypassed entirely and, in addition, even that blood not be made available amid such chaos:

'Direct admissions that bypass the already cluttered and overburdened emergency room are of utmost importance.....Blood and plasma are being removed from accident rooms, for the patient requiring these will not be released; he needs total care and the penetrating attention of experts' [5]

This trauma consultant dug the hole deeper by his less than helpful suggestion that, *'one might consider a hospital alert system which is sounded when such a patient gets to the front door'*.[5] That editorial writer appeared to side-step the question, among other crucial issues, as to what happened to the seriously injured before they reached the hospital. He came close to suggesting that care in any receiving area of a hospital be immediately determined by which specialty could best take care of the problem. Today's language would call that *'bar-code medicine.'* Needless to say, his opinions fortunately found no traction. Many who examined the problem of emergency care did so with a deeply entrenched bias born of a narrow focus constrained by their own specialty and expertise, or influenced by their overriding desire to maintain the status quo.[6] Seldom did clinicians and administrators examine the system of health care, but rather focused on the silos and segmented parts which largely were disconnected and dysfunctional.

If the inconvenience of the critically ill and injured were not enough, the sheer volume of patients added to the dilemma. To top it all off, who in their right mind would want to work in 'The Pit' a common moniker for the emergency room among students, residents and the institutional culture? Who indeed? As it stood, in the mid-twentieth century, not many practitioners were keen to take on such challenges. The emergency room of that era belonged to no one; it was more of an entry point to health care; often a last resort for the poor, disabled, and those with unanticipated medical catastrophes who happened to be in its general vicinity. The medical practitioners reflected the orphan nature of the place: ill-trained, often very junior members of a house staff, temporarily placed in this clinical setting which they simply tolerated and endured.

In the now-famous words of a Vietnam veteran surgeon who wrote in 1967, just after the exposé of the deficiencies in trauma care in America by the National Academy of Sciences.[8] (see Chapter 8):

'Wounded in the remote jungle or rice paddy of Vietnam, an American citizen has a better chance for quick definitive surgical care by board certified specialists than were he hit on a highway near his hometown in the continental United States. Even if he were struck immediately outside the emergency room of most United States hospitals rarely would he be given such prompt, expert operative care as routinely is furnished from the site of combat wounding in Vietnam.' [9]

Given the conditions existing in the emergency rooms of the sixties and seventies in many hospitals, it is little wonder that clinicians and administrators searched constantly for answers to this problem. The major challenge was not the physical space; that could fairly easily be expanded with better design, and equipment could be modernised. Often the focus was how to control the volume of patients being seen, some suggesting that patients be refused service if they presented with complaints considered to be trivial or clearly not emergencies. The recurring, and insurmountable, problem with this suggestion was that the analyses done giving rise to such a suggestion were retrospective, and assumed that a rash could be seen later, or fever in a child in most cases was not serious.[2] This was hardly reassuring if you were a worried parent.

Some consultants, specifically one representing the American Medical Association (AMA), suggested education was the key:

'The emergency department should treat only acute traumatic problems that require immediate medical attention. To do this, all persons involved,

129

especially members of the community the hospital serves, must be educated to this viewpoint.' [2]

It was evident that this advice would never fly. Not only did most patients present without trauma as their chief problem, patients never arrived with a diagnosis inscribed on their foreheads - and no bar codes. It would not be unlikely that a citizen with chest discomfort might well avoid seeking medical care after he had been informed that the emergency department treated only trauma cases. This could have disastrous consequences. In addition, blaming the victim failed to recognise that much of the problem was a system which offered few, if any, alternatives for accessing primary care

Emergency solutions

The plight of the emergency room of the fifties and sixties began to show some improvement by several innovative, if not revolutionary, developments beginning in 1961 and extending to the end of the decade.

The first was a plan for solving the problems of physician staffing developed in 1961 by Dr. Jim Mills in Alexandria, Virginia. It radically changed the way in which emergency care was delivered through their hospital to the Alexandria community. He decided to give up his private practice after recruiting three others to join him, and all four began staffing the emergency room 24 hours a day, seven days a week. As of June, 1961, for the first time in America, a hospital had a predictable, reliable, dedicated, well-trained and permanent staff to offer emergency care to their community. One of the first administrative details they attended to was to change the designation of their practice area from *'emergency room'* to *'emergency department.'* History was made. [10]

The *'Alexandria Plan'* and its initiators broke through the rigidly traditional structures that prevented improvements in the care offered to the unfiltered public who came for care. They did not stop there; they became the nidus around which congregated physicians and others of like mind who felt that the benefits of an organised group practice within an emergency *'department'* were so evident that a national dialogue should be encouraged. Slowly, over the course of the next decade, permanent staffing in the smaller hospitals became more and more common and gradually eroded the sceptical, if not hostile view of established medical staff of these community institutions. But change in the larger, and especially university-affiliated institutions remained slow. [11]

The second was the *'Belfast Experiment'* of 1966 [12] which demonstrated that life-saving care could be taken to the patient and systems developed based on the results of this bold initiative. No longer was emergency care wholly confined to a building or even to those who traditionally provided it. Perhaps the progressive attitude of Belfast could serve other places as well. Within months of the Belfast physicians' publication in the Lancet in 1967, an American cardiologist from St. Vincent's Hospital in Manhattan, William Grace, visited Geddes in Belfast, saw first-hand the system they had put in place, and within the year had established a similar model in the Greenwich Village area of New York.[13] The *'Belfast Experiment'* had emigrated to America.

The third cog in the revolutionary machinery was the creation of national associations dedicated to creating a new specialty: The American College of Emergency Physicians (1968),[14] the associations in the UK[15], Canada[16,17] and Australasia[18] each of which sought to organise and advocate the creation of a new medical specialty - emergency medicine. Convinced by their personal and professional experience that emergency rooms must be improved, especially with regard to the educational level and commitment of physicians working there, many physicians in the sixties organised locally for improved care and some even interested themselves in ambulance services.[19,20] Some of these physicians began to think beyond their local communities to a broader view of what might be accomplished with a national movement directed toward the same ends. In all four countries advocates reached that goal with the acceptance of emergency medicine as a fully accredited specialty with postgraduate training programmes that included defined curricula and licencing exams following formal education. Work towards defining the new specialty was rewarded with full Board status on the basis of the definition of the specialty agreed to by the credentialing group in each jurisdiction:

'A physician who specializes in Emergency Medicine focuses on the immediate decision-making and action necessary to prevent death or any further disability both in the pre-hospital setting by directing emergency medical technicians and in the emergency department. This specialist provides immediate recognition, evaluation, care, stabilization, and disposition of a generally diversified population of adult and pediatric patients in response to acute illness and injury.' [21]

The relatively rapid progress of emergency room practice becoming the specialty of emergency medicine occurred within a decade. Whereas most traditional specialties up to that time grew out of either a focus on increasing depth of understanding of diseases of various organs and

131

discoveries to combat them, or skilled techniques to diagnose and/or correct anatomical abnormalities, emergency medicine developed out of a desire by both the public and physicians to solve the problem of immediate care. There was a growing realisation that there had to be a species of specialist physician who could assess, triage and treat a broad spectrum of presenting complaints while managing serious injuries and illness, and at the same time directing the flow of patients either through the revolving door of the emergency department or into the care of the appropriate specialist.

Emergency medicine evolves

About the same time, the late sixties, the state of ambulance and accident services was unmasked and came under the blinding glare of the harsh criticism of the 'White Paper' from the National Academy of Sciences.[8] This field of growing importance helped define emergency medicine, although recognition of this fact was longer in coming than the official recognition of the specialty itself. The practice of delivering emergency care outside the confines of the hospital was identified by some visionaries as a type of clinical care unique to Emergency Medicine. It was unique in that it required the development of a system to deliver the care and, in all likelihood, surrogates (physician extenders) to deliver the care. This was quickly realised when the Belfast approach, with its doctor/nurse/ ambulance man team simply could not be sustained beyond the UK health system. This realisation led to the movement towards increased training of ambulance attendants reflecting the military model of 'corpsmen' or, as they began to be called in Vietnam, 'paramedics', The term most likely evolved from its military use designating a medic who parachutes in to rescue those in distress.[22] Government documents and the official curriculum designed by Nancy Caroline from the University of Pittsburgh was officially titled, 'National Training Course, Emergency Medical Technician, Paramedic.'[23]

Although early efforts, especially by progressive surgeons[24] and academic anaesthetists,[25,26] proposed the improvement of immediate pre-hospital care and suggested an increasing depth of involvement by physicians, it took the Belfast trial of out-of-hospital advanced cardiac care using sophisticated technology and drugs to prove the worth of early intervention by physicians in potentially catastrophic diseases.[26] In essence, the specialty of emergency medicine not only encompassed the emergency department, but also extended into the highways, byways and homes of communities. This component of medical service and approach to health care was unique to the new specialty and would expand significantly in the future. The lessons of Belfast were becoming the new normal. Indeed, the significant influence of the Belfast model in the development of pre-hospital care services has been widely recognised. In his invited oration on the occasion of the 2009 international conference in Belfast honouring Dr Pantridge and unveiling his portrait,[27,28] Richard Crampton of Virginia, one of the pioneers of the American version of the Pantridge/ Geddes model, paid tribute to the additional role that Pantridge played in establishing the specialty of emergency medicine:

'Feisty Frank revolutionised our emergency services in North America. He taught us to take care to the patient outside hospital. The Belfast system became the root and flower that crossed the Atlantic. It bloomed in and from North American casualty and emergency services.... Frank influenced North American emergency services from rural village general medical practices to sophisticated urban systems. Our independent hospital emergency or casualty departments did not exist until Frank ignited our North American firestorm in out-of-hospital care.' [28]

Following the creation by the American Board of Medical Specialties of the American Board of Emergency Medicine in 1979 [24] and the growing acceptance and popularity of the residency programmes for training physicians in the specialty, attention was directed to physician training in the field of *'pre-hospital'* emergency care. It was generally agreed that this aspect of an emergency system required involvement of physicians who were part and parcel of an emergency medical services system. Residency curricula have remained, however, inconsistent in their requirements as to the duration and type of exposure to out-of-hospital emergency and transport critical care.[30]

Early residency training

The work done by Drs. Safar and Benson, and the commitment and dedication of Phil Hallen and Gerald Esposito combined with Freedom House Enterprises to create one of the first broad-concept emergency medical services systems.[29,30] (see Chapter 8) It was one of the first staffed by physician-extenders or paramedics who were trained by a cadre of physicians, one of whom (Nancy Caroline) became nationally and internationally known for her work in curriculum development.[31-34] Following the creation of the Pittsburgh Emergency Medical Services Division of the Department of Public Safety, a new medical director and a graduate of the residency of the first university Department of Emergency Medicine, Dr. Ronald Stewart, arrived from Los Angeles in 1978 and began to build a broad programme shored up by a solid research base, an educational core and predictable funding to sustain it all. Chief among his goals was the establishment of a residency programme in the soon-to-be created specialty of emergency medicine. By the fall of 1978 an academic institute had been established[34] and within three years a residency with six candidates.

The plan for the education of residents in emergency medical services was one of the foundations of the curriculum, given the interaction Stewart had with Frank Pantridge and the familiarity he had with the Belfast model. Within the second year of residency training, residents were required to share 'radio call' with faculty members, monitor paramedic calls and to participate by driving to the scene when requested by the field team. A vehicle was provided to the resident(s) on call by the City of Pittsburgh EMS Division. The goal of this residency training requirement was not to supplement or intervene in care provided by paramedics; this happened only when the paramedic crew requested assistance or, in the judgement of the physician, more advanced intervention was required. Rather, it was to foster awareness and an appreciation in the physician trainee of the unique nature of out-of-hospital care and to connect emergency department clinical care with paramedic practice. Other benefits came of this arrangement: the strengthening of ties among members of the emergency team, whether in or out of the hospital setting, the opportunity for mutual education between physician staff/residents and field teams and for enhanced quality assurance. In addition, research projects and data collection were greatly enhanced by resident and faculty involvement.

The European Experience

In 1981, prompted by Douglas Chamberlain of Brighton, a self-appointed group of relevant specialists: Chamberlain(cardiology), Peter Baskett (anaesthesia), John McNae and Roger Sleet (emergency medicine), David Zideman (paediatric anaesthesia), Judith Fisher and Rodney Herbert (general practice) and Mark Harries (water life saving) met informally over drinks and founded the Community Resuscitation Advisory Group.[35] They later changed the title to the more impressive Community Resuscitation Council. With the backing of their various specialist organisations, and support from Laerdal Medical, they produced consensus guidelines. In 1984 this group became the Resuscitation Council UK [RC (UK)] and set about producing guidelines and organising scientific meetings with considerable success. By 1988 the RC(UK) felt that an effort should be made to unify the training and practice of resuscitation in all European countries. With this remit Chamberlain approached the European Society of Cardiology (ESC) to act as the parent body to a European Resuscitation Council, only to have the ESC turn down the proposal.[35] Undaunted , and once again over drinks, the core group of RC(UK) decided to forge ahead with a similar group of like minded European enthusiasts. This group, again supported by Laerdal Medical, met in Antwerp in 1988 and formed the European Resuscitation Council (ERC).[36] At the first executive committee meeting in August 1989, Peter Baskett was elected chairman – a position he held for five years.[37] Elsevier was approached to make the journal *Resuscitation* the official journal of the ERC, with Douglas Chamberlain as the first Editor-in-chief.[35]

By 1990, the ERC brought together the American Heart Association and the Resuscitation Councils of Australia, Latin America, New Zealand and South Africa to form the International Liaison Committee on Resuscitation (ILCOR).[38] The first meeting was held at the Utstein Abbey, near Stravanger, Norway in 1990 and resulted in a uniform system for reporting scientific studies on resuscitation – to be known as the Utstein Style. ILCOR set up Working Groups to address specific topics and produced internationally accepted guidelines on research methods, training and practice.[35,38]

In 1994, Frank Pantridge received honorary membership in the ERC – it's highest award.[39]

Putting it all together

As the decades have passed since the daring experiment of Pantridge and Geddes, improvements in the provision of emergency care have been widespread, and in the subspecialty of EMS, remarkably so. It is clear that the Belfast programme influenced the direction of both the nature and quality of immediate out-of-hospital emergency care. Unexpectedly perhaps, the tail began to wag the figurative dog when, as Dr. Crampton's tribute suggests, the fledgling specialty of Emergency Medicine was reinforced and further strengthened by the revolution in out-of-hospital emergency care.

We now focus on how the lessons learned from Belfast and beyond, served as the base for a major revolution in emergency care in a sea-bound corner of Canada on the rugged northeast coast of North America. It continues to serve as an example of how an emergency system, built on the foundations laid down over the first twenty-five years since Belfast, became a model of what could be done. (see Chapter 10)

References

1. Stevens R. Health care in the early 1960's. Health Care Financ Rev 1996;18:11-22.
2. Silver MH. The emergency department problem: an overview. JAMA 1966;198:146-9.
3. National Center for Health Statistics, Health, United States, 2012: with special feature on emergency care. Hyattsville, MD. 2013.
4. Moore GT, Bernstein R, Bonanno R. Effect of a neighborhood health center on hospital emergency room use. Med Care 1972;10:240-7.
5. Avellone JC. Emergency services for the severely injured (editorial). J Trauma 1965;5:436-7.
6. Walt AJ (editor). Panel: role of the specialist in the emergency room. J Trauma 1979; 19:481-91.
7. Casselbaum WH. Does the injured patient receive optimal care? J Trauma 1961;1:442-3.
8. Committee on Trauma, Shock and Anesthesia. Accidental death and disability: the neglected disease of modern society. Washington DC: National Academy of Sciences-National Research Council; Sept,1966.
9. Eiseman B. Combat casualty in Vietnam. J Trauma 1967;7:53-63.
10. Mills JD. A method of staffing a community hospital emergency department. Virginia Med Monthly. 1963; 90:518-9.
11. Merritt AK. The rise of emergency medicine In the sixties: paving a new entrance to the house of medicine. J Hist Med Allied Sc. 2014;69:251-93.
12. Pantridge JF, Geddes JS. Cardiac arrest after myocardial infarction. Lancet 1966; 807-8.
13. Grace WJ, Chadbourn JA. The mobile coronary care unit. Chest 1969; 55:452-5.
14. Suter R. Emergency medicine in the United States: a systemic review. World J Emerg Med 2012;3:5-10.
15. Sakr M, Wardrope J. Casualty, accident and emergency medicine, the evolution. J Accid Emerg Med. 2000; 17:314-9.
16. Elyas R. The birth of a new specialty: the history of emergency medicine in Canada. The proceedings of the 16th annual History of Medicine Days, 2007 Mar 30-31; Health Sciences Centre, Calgary, AB (Canada). c2007. p 277-86.
17. Walker DM. History and development of the Royal College specialty of emergency medicine. Ann RCPSC 1987; 20:349-52.
18. Maini A. History of Australasian emergency medicine [Internet]. Australasian College for Emergency Medicine; June 10, 2016 [accessed June 2017]. Available from: http://www.aemrounds.com/corecontent/2016/5/28/acem-origins.
19. Kelman HR, Lane DS. Use of the hospital emergency room in relation to use of private physicians. Am J Pub Health 1976; 66:1189-91.

20. Shortliffe EC, Hamilton TS, Noroian EH. The emergency room and the changing pattern of medical care. N Engl J Med 1958;258:20-5.
21. McSwain NE. Prehospital care from Napoleon to Mars: the surgeon's role. J Am Coll Surg. 2005; 200:487-504.
22. Farrington JD. Death in a ditch. Bull Am Coll Surg. 1967;52:121-30.
23. Caroline NL. National Training Course, Emergency Medical Technician, Paramedic. Dept. of Transportation, National Highway Traffic Safety Administration, 1977.
24. American Board of Medical Specialists. ABMS Guide to medical specialties 2017. Maryland Hts, MO: Elsevier: c2017. Emergency Medicine: p 9-10.
25. Page JO. The Paramedics. Morristown, NJ: Backdraft Publications; 1979.
26. Pantridge JF, Geddes JS: A mobile intensive-care unit in the management of myocardial infarction. Lancet 1967;2:271-3.
27. Evans AE. Frank Pantridge's Legacy: A symposium. Ulster Med J 2010;79(Suppl 1):3.
28. Crampton RS. Frank's legacy from a North American perspective. Ulster Med J 2010;79(Suppl 1):4-6
29. Safar P, Brose RA. Ambulance design and equipment for resuscitation. Arch Surg 1965;90:343-8.
30. Benson DM, Esposito G, Dirsch J, Whitney R, Safar P. Mobile intensive care by "unemployable" blacks trained as emergency medical technicians (EMT's) in 1967-69. J Trauma. 1972;12:409-21.
31. Katzer R, Cabanas G, Martin-Gill C. Emergency medical services education in emergency medicine residency programs: a national survey. Acad Emerg Med 2012;19:174-9.
32. Caroline NL. National Training Course, Emergency Medical Technician, Paramedic. Dept. of Transportation, National Highway Traffic Safety Administration, 1977.
33. Caroline NL. Will the real paramedic please stand up? Emerg Med Services 1977;6:16-18,85.
34. Stewart RD, Paris PM, Heller MB. Design of a resident in-field experience for an emergency medicine residency curriculum. (abstract) Ann Emerg Med 1985;14:491.
35. Baskett PJF. Douglas Chamberlain – a man for all decades of his time. Resuscitation 2007;72:344-9.
36. Nolan J, Chamberlain D, Soar J, Parr M, Zorab J. Peter Baskett – 40 years as a resuscitation leader and mentor. Resuscitation 2008;77:279-82.
37. Chamberlain DA. The European Resuscitation Council. Resuscitation 1992;24:99-101.
38. Chamberlain DA. The International Liason Committee on Resuscitation (ILCOR) – past and present. Resuscitation 2005;67:157-61.
39. Baskett PJF. Citation for J. Frank Pantridge MC, CBE, MD, FRCP for honorary membership of the European Resuscitation Council. Resuscitation 1994;28:183-4.

Chapter 10

Putting it all together: development of the Nova Scotia emergency medical services system

After the proven success of extending advanced emergency treatment outside the fixed confines of the hospital, clinicians were challenged on several fronts. One of the first, and perhaps the most important, was who should provide the care - ambulance drivers? public safety personnel? nurses? physicians? The answer to this crucial question appeared, in part at least, out of the tragedy and fog of 20th century wars: World Wars I and II, the Korean conflict and Vietnam. Although World War I saw attempts to deploy soldiers trained in initial care to the trenches, most of the wounded had to be transported from forward aid posts to Casualty Clearing Stations located to the rear, but transport times could be long and as dangerous for the care-givers as for the wounded.[1] Out of that war came evidence of the value of blood replacement, the influence of time on survival and the principle of triage - the sorting of casualties. But improvements in care of the wounded and the use of physician extenders to provide immediate battlefield care and rapid transport by air came out of military conflicts later in the century. From the Vietnam war came the name 'paramedic' borrowed likely from earlier parachute medics but commonly applied to the combat medic who became the physician extender providing advanced battlefield care in that conflict. These changes profoundly influenced the direction of emergency care on the home front [2], culminating in these three defining developments of the past fifty years:

1. The recognition of the need for improvement of the care of trauma patients, both inside and outside the hospital.[2]
2. The provision of advanced care outside hospital for those suspected of suffering acute myocardial infarction and other cardiovascular diseases.[3]
3. The creation of a new medical specialty, emergency medicine and its subspecialty, emergency medical services (EMS).[4]

Since that first successful Belfast programme however, it has not always been easy to duplicate the system those clinicians put in place.

Communities and medical facilities in other countries or even in nearby neighbourhoods differed, sometimes widely, in respect to what resources were at hand and the leadership required to improve the system. As we have seen, out-of-hospital care was primitive in most jurisdictions; ambulance service varied widely in quantity and quality, and lines were rigidly drawn as to who did what and to whom . The reasons for this primitive state of out-of-hospital emergency care are rooted, in part, in the fact that health and medical care became almost exclusively the domain of institutions, particularly hospitals, less so physicians' offices or community clinics. This trend had been recognised earlier in the fifties and the sixties by both administrators and clinicians.[3,4] The pre-hospital care of trauma victims and of other life-threatening emergencies became the focus of only a few clinicians and physician researchers prior to the work of Pantridge and Geddes.[6,7]

Progress towards improvement of ambulance services and pre-hospital care was made more difficult by the apathy or, in some cases, opposition of medical leaders and by others already entrenched in the health system. Even in the late 20th century there appeared to be wide variations in the quality of care offered and scant attention paid to the scope of care outside institutions.

Despite government-funded universal health plans in Canada , very little attention was given to ambulance and paramedic services and fifty years later several of these same jurisdictions require user fees for emergency care and transport.[7] This curious lack of consistency could be a holdover from when medical or health care was considered to be the domain of institutions and those who work in and govern them, and anything else was of little importance. The Belfast experience changed that; physicians were convinced of the need for the provision of early advanced care, and that a system could be developed outside the hospital to do that. Even now, few realise the scope and quality of the services provided by modern and well-run emergency medical service and therefore tend to be unaware of its importance or how much the public depends on it working well. The administration of such health services by agencies outside the health care system (i.e. fire, police or governmental) could lead the public to believe emergency medical services is not a crucial part of a continuum of care, but separate and distinct from the health system.

As with the law and other aspects of social engagement, many of our decisions in health care reflect *precedents*; what has been successful before, demonstrated either in formal research protocols or our careful experience and observations in our own practice. Unfortunately for practitioners in

139

evolving systems, the evaluation may be tedious and slow in enabling even minor changes designed to improve the system of health care delivery. It is even more difficult to make those changes when a system is already entrenched, rigidly defined, and, without any in-depth examination, appears to be working quite well.

The ideal situation would be to initiate reform in a system or jurisdiction in which very few rigid rules or protocols were already in place but, with strong leadership, clearly-defined goals and a blueprint as to how to reach them, improvements could be made and those goals achieved. In other words, those who start later on the road to reform have the advantage of having the way if not paved, at least the potholes filled in. Such an opportunity of major EMS reform occurred some twenty-five years after the landmark Belfast paper [8] and about fifteen years after the designation of Emergency Medicine as a specialty in the United States and Canada. In 1993 a concerted effort was launched to institute a major reform of emergency services in the eastern Canadian province of Nova Scotia. What resulted was a case study of what could be achieved, and what missteps might occur in a comprehensive plan not merely to improve emergency services, but to cement them into the bedrock of a reformed health care structure. The experience and solid grounding which had been gained from others' pioneering efforts over the twenty years before this reform was introduced were crucial in forging an EMS system almost from the pavement up.

The Laboratory

The Canadian province of Nova Scotia clings tenuously to North America by a narrow, low-lying isthmus, Chignecto, connecting it to the main landmass of the continent. At its narrowest point the isthmus is twenty-four kilometres wide and if sea levels were to rise twelve metres, Nova Scotia would consist of two larger islands- the north (current) island of Cape Breton and the mainland of the province. Despite having the second-smallest land mass (55,000 km^2) of the ten provinces and three northern territories of Canada, Nova Scotia has a ragged and jagged coastline of almost ten thousand kilometres with an estimated four thousand coastal and lake islands, three thousand lakes and cut through by hundreds of rivers and streams. The terrain of the province is a mix of rolling forested hills, lush valleys, deep coves and coastal islands, giving rise to lofty stubs of ancient mountains in the sparsely-populated North Highlands of Cape Breton. Most of the population lives within a forty-minute drive from the capital region of Halifax, the rest in towns and

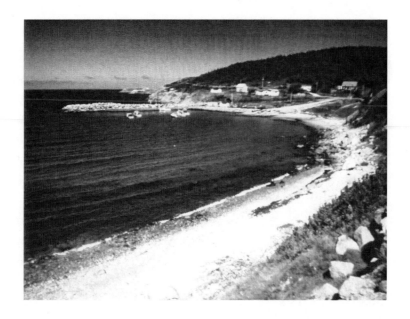

Figure 10.1 Nova Scotia is Canada's second-smallest province but has a coastline of 10,000 km, with small villages clinging to cliffs and outcroppings. Roads can be treacherous and travel slow.

villages scattered around the rugged coastline with farms in the interior valleys and low-rising forested hills. (Figure 10.1)

With a recent surge in immigration, the population of the province totals 953,000, Halifax region has a growing population of over 403,000 (2016). In large measure due to its history of early European colonisation Nova Scotia is home to ten degree-granting universities and a Community College system with thirteen campuses and twenty-five thousand students. There is one medical school, Dalhousie University Faculty of Medicine with one campus in Halifax and one in Saint John in the neighbouring province of New Brunswick. Several of these universities and other diploma colleges provide training for other health professionals.

The province is served by a series of four-lane (divided) highways with fair-to-good secondary roads connecting coastal towns and villages with fifty-four collaborative primary care clinics, small rural hospitals and regional hospital facilities. This network of health centres feeds via the highway system into the single tertiary-care centre for the province composed of the IWK Health Centre (Children's and Women's Hospitals) and the Queen Elizabeth II Health Sciences Centre. These tertiary care facilities are teaching sites of the Dalhousie University Faculties of Medicine, Health and Dentistry. Patients are transported from local outlying health facilities by the Emergency Health Services (EHS) paramedic ground ambulances, or, depending on medical need, by special Critical Care Transport Units or by the EHS Lifeflight helicopter/fixed-wing service.

Health care, including physician and other approved professional services are funded by the Department of Health and Wellness, this government ministry and minister being responsible to the Legislative Assembly through the Cabinet, chosen from the party with the most seats in the Assembly, its leader named the Premier. The health system of the province is, as in all Canadian provinces, required to fulfill the defined principles of the Canada Health Act of 1984[9] in order to receive partial funding from the national government. Those basic principles include:

1. **Universality** - all residents of the province are entitled to health care under uniform terms.
2. **Portability** - insurance coverage, beginning after three months residency status, is valid in all provinces and territories and when traveling abroad.
3. **Public administration** - the insurance plan of a province must be administered on a non-profit basis by a public authority.
4. **Accessibility** - reasonable access to all medically necessary hospital and physician services must not be impeded by financial or other barriers.
5. **Comprehensiveness** - all medically necessary services must be insured by each provincial plan and no extra-billing by physicians or other health professionals for these services is permitted.

In addition, each province provides insurance coverage for prescribed pharmaceuticals; plans vary as to coverage - all plans cover senior citizens over sixty-five and usually those on public assistance and other selected groups, depending on the province.

The current network of EMS services and the current transport system are a result of relatively rapid changes in both organisation and facilities which were begun in the mid-nineties and are celebrated in this the 20th anniversary year of major EMS reform.These improvements in out-of-hospital care not only laid down the basis of the current system, but they were also designed to carry through a planned process in expectation of future correction, expansion and further reforms. This remaking of the underfunded and largely unsupported ambulance system that existed in Nova Scotia before 1993, may be regarded as an example of the often difficult process required to establish a modern, evidence-based and medically-accountable EMS system.

The way we were

In respect to out-of-hospital emergency care, the province of Nova Scotia fared no better than the sad state of affairs described by the American review of ambulance services published in 1966.[10] In fact, the state of affairs might have been worse than those described in the NRC report, with the added challenges of North Atlantic winters and, prior to 1955, the thorny problem of the rail and automobile ferry service connecting the northern island of Cape Breton (a major industrial production centre of coal and steel) with the Nova Scotia mainland. Winters made quick work of ferry schedules and, combined with winds and currents passing through the Canso Strait even on a good day, added a dangerous element to the inconvenience of travelers as well as isolating the northern island for days at a time. Following the opening of the Canso Causeway in August of that year, travel to the tertiary care centres in Halifax was markedly improved.

In contrast to out-of-hospital emergency care available elsewhere, the public of the province was well served in most instances by the reputable and dedicated members of the St. John's Ambulance, whose presence at large gatherings and teaching of first-aid was popular and widely appreciated by the community. The Canadian Red Cross and the Boy Scouts' and Girl Guides' Associations were heavily involved in teaching basic first-aid as well as offering help in mass casualty situations or local calamities. But as with other jurisdictions both in Canada, the United States and overseas, there was no regionalised system of ambulances with trained personnel. Other than transport vehicles of various types offered by large corporate entities for their workers, especially in mining areas, ambulances prior to the seventies were of varied design which could, at best, be described as a motley collection of funeral hearses, station wagons or worse. To be fair, this was little different from most other jurisdictions, at least until the decade of the seventies saw ambulance operators in the province form the Ambulance Operators Association of Nova Scotia (AOANS). Efforts during and beyond that decade were made by this group to interest government in a publicly-subsidised system. Their frequent pleas fell on deaf political ears, and little progress was made, except for attempts by the Association to enforce standards set largely by the association with no backing in law. Not only did no legislation support their efforts, but the lack of funding allowed for only the most meagre policing of what regulations actually existed. This resulted in spotty service and a debilitating sense of frustration on the part of the leaders and many of the members of the Association. Their cause did not die, but it stuttered along wounded until the decade of the nineties, during which their goals were to be realised.

The state of pre-hospital emergency services in the province was not much better or worse than hospitals provided throughout the province. House calls by physicians were still quite common, especially in rural areas, and the value of early intervention in even serious conditions was unrecognised. Nova Scotia in the decade of the sixties, and until a regionalised health system was developed in the nineties, had forty-eight hospitals scattered throughout the province - largely independent of each other. Standards and regulations were largely developed locally, with some consultation with the Department of Health in Halifax. Each was governed by a local board with many members appointed by the Minister of Health, and each Board governed by unique bylaws. The tertiary care facilities, located in the capital region of Halifax, differed in both size and specialty services, and even large hospitals there were independent in governance and budget from each other. Two large teaching hospitals in the city, no more than two blocks separate, duplicated several programmes and had separate medical staffs (although some had privileges in both). The Halifax Infirmary was founded in 1886 by the Sisters of Charity and was considered the GP (General Practice) hospital; the Victoria General, dating from 1859 as the City and Provincial hospital, was more closely associated with Dalhousie University's Health faculties. Both offered emergency room care, with varying physician staffing patterns and length of tenure. The hospitals in the province ranged in size from the smallest with eight beds in the North Highlands area of the province, to the large Dalhousie medical school teaching hospitals in Halifax, with hundreds of beds and specialty training (residency) programmes.

The sometimes-frustrating struggle of some physicians to establish emergency medicine as a specialty in the American House of Medicine appeared to be less strained in Canada and elsewhere, perhaps because the ground had been already tilled in America. (see Chapter 9) Efforts in the province of Nova Scotia to improve both in-hospital and pre-hospital care were much less dramatic and rested on the shoulders of a few clinicians who were quite aware of the forces gathering momentum south of the Canada-USA border. They took note particularly of the efforts to develop academic programmes for specialty training. Although the Ambulance Operators Association of Nova Scotia proposed minimum standards for ambulances and attendants and made early efforts to define a curriculum, government was unresponsive even into the 1980s and subsidies were held at a very low level.[11]

Emergency rooms in the province during the sixties were largely receiving areas reserved for unexpected accidents or for those unfortunate citizens in extremis from a variety of maladies. Clinical coverage for all but the large hospitals was, as elsewhere, assigned to a nurse on duty who might call the patient's physician or accost the first MD passing by. In the coalfields of the province where British companies operated mines, 'check off' systems of insurance were developed as early as 1883 and perhaps earlier. Under this system, miners were obliged to have an amount (usually forty to fifty cents) deducted from each pay stub to reimburse physicians and sustain hospitals within the community.[12] This resulted in greater stability of hospitals and reliability of physician coverage. Pre-hospital care was largely in the form of house calls and, in the event of mining accidents or emergencies in the steel mills, physicians were expected to go to the scene.

The improvement of in-hospital and out-of-hospital emergency care in Nova Scotia began subtly in the early to mid-sixties when the decision was made by the administration of the Victoria General Hospital and the University to offer the directorship of the emergency room to an experienced general surgeon with a certificate in orthopaedics. His name was Robert Scharf, and he had acquired the reputation of being a superb teacher with a talent for engaging students and residents and carrying them along with his enthusiasm for medicine.(Figure 10.2)

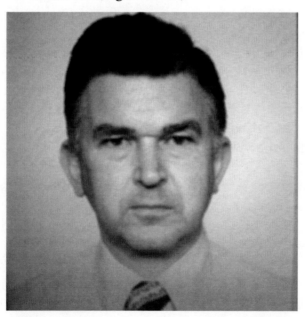

Figure 10.2 Dr. Robert Scharf (1924-2007) was the first full-time director of the Halifax University teaching hospital and organised the first ambulance training courses in the early sixties. As early as 1968 he was petitioning the Royal College in Canada for emergency medicine to be credentialed as specialty.

145

Robert Scharf had already taken an interest in the ambulance services and the teaching of attendants both at the hospital and in his own community.[13] His management style resembled his approach to teaching - direct, precise, but skilfully diplomatic. His approach to administration was straightforward and transparent; his decisions were never murky, his opinions clear and sometimes starkly stated. He was a leader. His teaching style was welcomed especially by medical and nursing students who would be coaxed into giving an opinion or gently encouraged to answer a question or suggest what a shadow on an X-ray might be, or some other such medical mystery. He had an egalitarian approach to instruction, adjusting that approach to fit the learner's role in health care, a teaching strategy which endeared him especially to ambulance personnel, who were unaccustomed to being included in teaching sessions or, even less likely to have sessions designed specifically for them.

The arrival of Robert Scharf sparked an interest in several students as they progressed through their final years of medical school as they were heading out, usually to practice in local communities before deciding on a specialty residency. His infectious enthusiasm for his work in emergency medicine was contagious, and that enthusiasm encompassed his eclectic interests in ambulance services including the appropriate design of equipment and vehicles *('ambulances should look like bread trucks- not Cadillacs!')* as well as the training levels of attendants. By the end of the sixties, at least one of his disciples (RDS) had committed to returning to the Victoria General following two or three years of general practice in a remote area of the North Highlands of Nova Scotia and promised to consider specialty training focused on emergency medicine. Within a year Scharf had discovered the single academic programme with a full residency in what was to become, but was not yet, the specialty of emergency medicine. It was located at the Los Angeles County-University of Southern California Medical Centre, over 6,400 km from the door of the cottage hospital in which Bob Scharf's former student was finishing up his first two years of community general practice. Together they would take their careers in similar directions to grasp the challenge of changing for the better the *'safety net of the health care system.'* But to do that, both would have to take a detour south, survive amid a tangle of freeways and veil of smog, and eventually land back where they started almost two decades later.

Southern detour

Ron Stewart's journey in his Volvo station wagon from the North Highlands of his beloved island of Cape Breton took six days to navigate the thousands of kilometres before arriving amid the snaking chaos of what was the Los Angeles freeway system. He had been only once to the city, having flown into LAX for his interview after which he was accepted for the last opening in the second-year of the new residency at *'Big County'*, more formally, *The University of Southern California-Los Angeles County Hospital, Department of Emergency Medicine*. Coming from a small cottage hospital of about twelve beds in the fishing village of Neil's Harbour (population 242) along the northern coast of Cape Breton, he found himself navigating the eight lanes of the westbound Interstate 10 leading, so he thought, to Big County. It did not go well. Never having seen the giant hospital from ground level, he did manage to take the right exit, but turned left instead of right, and mistook the Sears Building in East Los Angeles for the hospital. A rather bemused (and armed) security guard promptly directed him out of the Ladies Lingerie department (it was immediately inside the main entrance), to the correct address northward on the same street.[14]

The culture shock of having gone from a hospital which saw one thousand patients a *year* to a department which saw one thousand patients a *day* wore off quickly with help from colleagues and new-found friends, but not without the odd misstep or two. Not having used a single-line dial phone for three years or so, it was a luxury which he felt went unappreciated by his colleagues - a fact which the ersatz Canadian mentioned to his puzzled colleagues as he wondered how blasé some people could be about the conveniences of modern life and living. The pace of the department, the unreality of the Jail Ward, the mix of accents and languages from both staff and patients, and the sudden introduction to the *'L.A. Scene'* added to the challenge of cultural adjustment, to put it mildly.

The department was the only academic Department of Emergency Medicine in the world as of July 1972, and the second emergency medicine residency. The department was, for the eager and young physician from the north, a cauldron bubbling over with possibilities and opportunities. Early on in his time, Stewart focused on the role of physician extenders both inside and outside the hospital. A programme of training Physician Assistants (PAs) was particularly intriguing. Many of these employees of the department were former military *'corpsmen'* (or *'paramedics'* as they were dubbed in Vietnam) and had extensive clinical experience in triage, as well as in trauma assessment and management. Residents in the department often looked to PAs for practical instruction in casting, suturing and the other many surgical procedures performed in one of the busiest department's divisions - 'Minor Trauma'. In addition, he became equally fascinated by a programme which extended advanced emergency care outside the hospital, the Los Angeles County Paramedic Program, begun the previous year by several cardiologists who were inspired by the work of Pantridge and Geddes.[8,15] He assumed a major role in developing the curricula of both programmes, and within two years had been appointed the first Medical Director of the Paramedic Training Institute of Los Angeles County. (see Chapter 8)

At the invitation of the Chair of the Department, Dr. Gail Anderson, Stewart decided to remain in place following the completion of his residency as an Assistant Professor and to continue his role in heading up the rapidly-expanding Paramedic Institute and to help shore up the residency. He resigned himself to remaining in Los Angeles, rather than returning home, because the Royal College, the governing body of the specialties in Canada, had not yet approved Emergency Medicine as a specialty and there would be no academic positions likely available. So the plans of Scharf and Stewart were put on indefinite hold. Soon after, however, the Department of Emergency Medicine suffered a blow when its popular and talented Residency Director, Robert Dailey, left to develop an emergency medicine programme in the Central Valley region of California. Despite the quality of the residents, the residency was left leaderless and vulnerable, and Stewart felt he knew of only one person who could possibly fill the shoes of the departing Dr. Dailey. That person was his former mentor and now close friend, Robert Scharf of his alma mater Dalhousie Medical School in Halifax, Nova Scotia. The plan that had been hatched some years earlier in Halifax took a southern detour as Bob Scharf reunited with his former student and now colleague; but while the ultimate plan of returning northward was put on hold, it was not forgotten by either of them. Bob Scharf accepted the Residency Director's position and became a valuable member of the teaching staff, as well as a major proponent of specialty status for emergency medicine as he had been in Canada several years earlier.

Northern retreat

Despite his dedication and profound commitment to the people and rapidly expanding initiatives in emergency medicine in Los Angeles, Stewart felt he needed a smaller and more academically related programme with a solid research and educational base. An offer from the University

148

of Pittsburgh came through one of the gurus in resuscitation medicine, Dr. Peter Safar. The university was looking for a Director for the university hospital's emergency department and the Mayor of the city was looking for a Director of EMS; the two positions were combined. After the usual interviews, and with some reluctance, Stewart left for Pittsburgh in 1978 to continue what became a decade-long trek across the continent and back home to Nova Scotia.[16]

On arriving in the city that would be his home for a full decade, the newly appointed Medical Director of Pittsburgh EMS found himself almost perpetually surprised; a solid EMS system was in place and built on the work done by several of his 'heroes of EMS'- Caroline, Safar, Benson, Freedom House and others. (see Chapter 8) The city itself was a wonderful mix of diverse neighbourhoods, blue-collar work ethic with stellar academic institutions and it was undergoing an exciting transformation from an industrial city to a high-tech giant. And the welcome was beyond anything he might have expected.

Within a year real progress had been made towards putting in place the building blocks of an emergency medicine structure - an exercise which, a decade later, would prove to be invaluable training for the major challenges which awaited across the border in Nova Scotia. A research and teaching institute was established, The Center for Emergency Medicine, with leadership from the University and other major teaching hospitals in the city. A residency programme in Emergency Medicine started with six original, recruits, headed by a dynamic residency director - a son of Pitt's medical school, Dr. Paul Paris, who had trained in Maine and Los Angeles. The birth of The Center and the residency helped support the already solid EMS system, a third-service agency of the City government. These were the salad days of Emergency Medicine in the city and, for many of those involved, represented an almost-golden era of expansion, exciting research and unlimited optimism. (see Chapter 8)

The early work by Scharf to convince the Royal College of Physicians and Surgeons in Canada to embrace the specialty of emergency medicine bore fruit following Dr. Scharf's return to Canada from Los Angeles in 1976. Within several years of his return, the College began formal preparations to add the specialty of Emergency Medicine to its roster, and with that the way was clear for the Canadian nomad to fix his sight on the north star and head towards the salt air of the North Atlantic. With the help yet again of his mentor, he had come full circle and he could now go home.

One more stop

The city of Toronto is as 'foreign' to most Atlantic Canadians as the Antarctic. But to the medical nomad's surprise again, it was not at all foreign. Quite the opposite. The city and the University hospitals became very much a medical home, or at the very least a very welcoming detour on his way east. The EMS system of the city was highly developed and personnel were extremely well trained, professional and totally committed to doing a good job. The University's Sunnybrook hospital housed the busiest and most organised trauma centre in the country, and research was well advanced. Far from being just 'a clean L.A.' as someone once called it, Toronto offered superb clinical exposure in emergency medicine and the potential for significant research, if only by virtue of the numbers and the infrastructure already in place.

Especially valuable was the experience gained from the highly organised trauma network backed up by the provincial air ambulance service which reflected the similarly high-quality paramedic EMS service of Toronto and area EMS. The lessons of regionalised trauma services were embedded in the mind and notebook of the inveterate Nova Scotian who soon headed eastward.

Home again

The Victoria General Hospital and Dalhousie Medical School in 1989 were not the same as he had left them almost twenty years earlier. His mentor and friend Bob Scharf had retired back home to Nova Scotia from the Saint John Regional Hospital in the neighbouring province of New Brunswick. The Emergency Room at the Halifax Victoria General was now an 'Emergency Department' staffed by well-trained and full-time emergency physicians with first-class leadership, at least three of whom had formal residency training and several more were expected. The Emergency Department came under the administrative management of the Department of Anaesthesia of the hospital and therefore of the University. But change was on the way, and within several years an autonomous Division under the Dean's office was created, and although this conferred a slice of self-directed independence, it did not guarantee a decision-making role in budgetary or policy initiatives; only a full academic department could do that. A full decade was required to reach Departmental status (in 1998), a tribute to the enlightened and skilled leadership current at that time, aided by a sympathetic Dean and equally sympathetic, conspiratorial and reformist Health Minister.

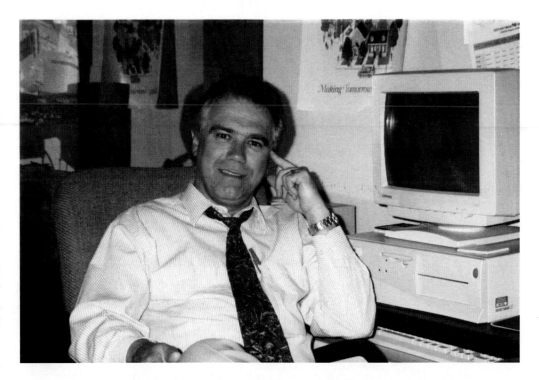

Figure 10.3 Dr. Michael Murphy was appointed EMS Commissioner in 1994 to effect a complete revamping of the ambulance service and to plan the educational programmes to support the reformed system. He was qualified in both emergency medicine and anaesthesia.

A major force in the development and leadership in Emergency Medicine and EMS at Dalhousie and the Victoria General was Dr. Michael Murphy, who assumed the directorship of the Emergency Department and much later the Department of Anaesthesia as well.(Figure 10.3) Trained in Emergency Medicine at the Denver General programme of Dr. Peter Rosen, he returned to Canada, along with several other Canadians and completed his qualification in anaesthesia. He was thus a perfect fit for the Emergency Department which, at the time, was located within the Department of Anaesthesia. He worked closely with a colleague, Doug Sinclair, who was later to rise high in the ranks of emergency medicine, the medical school and later hospital administration. Dr. Stewart hoped to do clinical work in the department and transplanted his laboratory from Sunnybrook, along with several other research projects in acute airway management. His lab work was focused on the effect of molecular coating of several drugs in a preparation for topical application and inhalation as a means of convenient and rapid emergency administration and local anaesthesia.[17]

151

Stewart's work in the Emergency Department at the Victoria General Hospital was exactly what he was looking for and it proved to be both satisfying and rewarding, not only for the clinical patient contact but also for the opportunity of restoring former friendships and cultivating new ones. His work became, for him, an ideal balance between his research lab and airway projects, his shift work in the Emergency Department and his growing involvement in medical student teaching. Because the Department was officially under the Department of Anaesthesia, Stewart had a foot in both camps, giving him the opportunity to develop formal and informal ties to anaesthesia colleagues and several projects in analgesia and sedation that could be useful to emergency medicine procedure and practice. With the help of Murphy, during these introductory years he forged a particularly close collegial relationship with one of Anaesthesia's young researchers, Dr. Orlando Hung, just back from a two-year Fellowship at Stanford. Stewart had brought with him from Pittsburgh the design of a new 'Lightwand' airway device which caught the eye and interest of Hung who began clinical trials with the new device as well as expanding the scope of the liposomal studies.[18,19] Because of these similar research interests, particularly in the management of airway problems, the two began a collaboration which flourished for twenty-five years and has continued in full vigour.[20]

One of the legacies of Bob Scharf during his years at the Victoria General was the efforts he made to include hospital-based ambulance attendants in his teaching. He quickly designed 'Ambulance Training Courses' which he held frequently, sometimes in his home. These were later credentialed and as medical students in the sixties we were frequently quite jealous of these early paramedics who knew far more about what to do at the scene of an accident or sudden illness than ever we did as interns and certainly as medical students. Although interns assigned to the emergency room in the sixties at Dalhousie were required to go out on the ambulance on major calls, at a scene the MDs were almost totally dependent on the skilled ambulance attendants and learned fast that things were very different 'out there'- something which stuck with most of them for the duration of their careers.(Figure 10.4) While in the Department in Los Angeles, Stewart had recalled his experiences with these early paramedics and he credits their influence as paramount in his decision to focus on physician-extenders during his time in the Los Angeles residency and beyond, and focused his career on their crucial role and their education in emergency medicine and EMS.

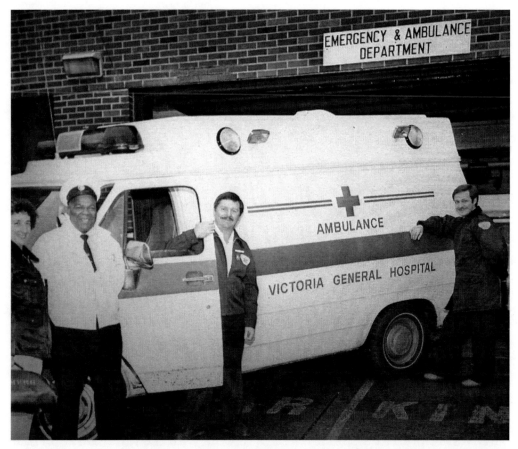

Figure 10.4 During the 1960s interns assigned to the Emergency Department at the Victoria General Hospital, Halifax were required to accompany ambulance attendants on emergency calls. They were to be 'taught rather than get in the way' as Dr. Scharf defined their role. This was later influential in the Pittsburgh residency system.

As his research progressed into the nineties and his circle of colleagues and friends in Nova Scotia widened, his distress increased at seeing the gaps in the health care system as he understood them. The idea of advanced life support and an extended role for ambulance attendants on which he based much of his research and career in the United States appeared to be stalled at best, dismissed at worst. Dismissed perhaps by most decision-makers in the health system, but accompanied by a growing interest - and frustration - by ambulance personnel, the Ambulance Operators Association and the increasing numbers of emergency physicians in the major hospitals. But before this could possibly happen, the basic system required of any modern EMS system had to be shored up and, in some cases, created. Even at the beginning of the final decade of the 20th century Nova Scotia did not have any coherent system of ambulance services with predictable

153

funding and had no 'home' in the Ministry of Health. It was devoid of any legislated standards or regulations and had very little physician oversight, save for several dedicated volunteers who were committed to doing their part, however small they felt it was, to make things better.

But with this realisation came the conviction that in order to accomplish what would probably be a major task - the implementation of a modern emergency medical services system with all the supports and elements required to make it work - it would be necessary for Stewart not only to raise awareness of the lack of services and the necessity for reform, but also to step up and, horrors of horrors, put his name on a ballot.

The way we were

Canada doesn't have only one health care system, it has thirteen. That is, under the country's constitution, the provision of health services is the responsibility of the Ministries of Health of the ten provincial and three territorial governments. With a looming election for the provincial parliament on the horizon and likely in 1993, political parties began preparation of their platforms for presentation during the expected campaign. Looming also was the stated intention of the national government to reduce the size of transfer payments that were part of the Canadian policy of equalisation in its federal system. The challenge of any party was to present a plan for 'health reform' with the full realisation that federal monies were going to shrink and 'doing more with less' would soon become the mantra of political and public life.

Following the provincial election in 1993 of a reformist liberal government by a hefty majority (40 of 52 seats in the Legislative Assembly) the general changes announced during the election campaign had to be fashioned into a practical approach to implementing the system reform promised in the party platform. Having been elected as the Member of the Legislative Assembly (MLA) for Cape Breton North, Stewart was appointed Minister of Health and would now have the opportunity and the responsibility to implement his plans for reformed emergency health care in the province. It was soon apparent that to accomplish the desired changes, the major components of the system could not be disturbed without jeopardising the whole structure. The centralised nature of health governance, entrusted to the Department (Ministry) of Health, allowed for relatively efficient analysis and planning, if not rapid initiation of changes on the ground. But there needed to be a safety net.

Before the actual election, the general priorities outlined in preparation of the future government's platform focused on:

- Changes in the governance and services offered by hospitals in the province.
- Expansion of home care/home hospital services to all citizens, not only to certain groups.
- Expansion of the role of nurses and other health professionals in the system.
- Promotion of research with the creation of an agency or foundation.
- Restructuring of health services under four or five regional health units rather than 50+ hospital boards.
- Restructuring of the province's Pharmacare programme.
- Introduction of a tobacco control programme and the legislation required to reduce the toll of the addiction.
- Creation of an Emergency Health Services division of the ministry for the platform for the major reform of the system.*

These changes, not listed in order of priority, were to be implemented over the four to five-year government mandate, priorities being determined not only by the looming fiscal reality but rather by the perceived urgency for these changes or improvements. It was agreed that, in respect to health services offered, priority needed to be given to ensuring that a 'safety net' was in place especially as the role and programmes of hospitals were altered. That safety net was a newly-designed and extensively renewed 'Emergency Health Services' initiative that would form the base upon which were anchored the health system changes which followed.

Within months of Stewarts' appointment as the new Minister in the Department of Health the plans for revision and renewal of emergency health services within the province began to unfold. Several solid planks in the process of health reform were already in place. One was The Provincial Health Council, formed several years earlier under the leadership of Ms. Mary Jane Hampton, an articulate and talented health consultant, who early on was tasked with developing needed changes in the health system. Unfortunately the Council was given little clout, but served admirably to tap into the opinions of communities as they articulated their needs by means of public meetings, petitions and study groups.

* The decision to use the term 'Emergency Health Services'(EHS) rather than 'Emergency Medical Services' (EMS) was debated at some length, the Minister arguing that the plan for trained personnel (paramedics) for an eventual expanded role should be linked to health services broadly and not only within the context of ambulance or emergency services as EMS usually implies.

The Council was the model for a Minister's committee appointed to draw up a definitive plan, a blueprint as to how to achieve the government's goals, already announced through Legislature debates and Ministerial directives. Ms. Hampton became the Director of Health Reform in the new government and the Blueprint Committee was chaired by Dr. David MacLean, a health policy and public health expert, who in 1994 was still associated with the World Health Organisation. Independent of this Blueprint Committee, planning groups within the Ministry (Department of Health) were set up to examine the current state of ambulance services in the province and to recommend to the Minister the structure, policies and implementation strategies of a reformed regionalised emergency health services system.

To achieve these ends, it was clear that the leadership delegated to steer the unwieldy ship around the shoals and tempests of a complete reform required patience, clear-headedness, credibility in the field of emergency care and financial wizardry of the like not usually seen in health professionals. The decision was to ensure there would be solid medical input into the design, but also that the proposed system was affordable and, although a significant budget increase was anticipated, it would be crafted by firm and experienced hands. The Minister chose for this significant role Dr. Michael Murphy, with a stellar background and formal training in both specialties of emergency medicine and anaesthesia, and Ms. Ann Petley-Jones, a well-known local financial administrator and a consultant known for genteel diplomacy, intelligence and also for her quiet but gritty determination. After some months of debate and political to-ing and fro-ing,[21] the legislation required for creating an Emergency Health Services system was passed by the provincial parliament and proclaimed as law in June of 1994.

The decision by the Commissioner and ministerial staff that once the general principles and direction of the revamping of the EHS system were outlined, a 'blueprint' for implementing the changes would be analysed and possibly revised by a panel of invited specialists in emergency care. These consultants would be international in scope, mainly from Canada, the United Kingdom, Australia and the United States. Their report served Mike Murphy well in preparing several submissions to the Minister, the main one delivered in 1994 and known usually as *The Murphy Report*.[22] The report was withering and definitive in its criticism of the then-system, but it laid out the blueprint for a major overhaul in the areas of ambulances, legislation, organisation, programmes and training; the timing and progress of change, it cautioned, would be dependent on budgetary considerations.[23]

Reflecting the importance that the government felt Emergency Health Services played in the health system as a whole and the reform strategy in particular, the budget for the ministry was realigned to accommodate the significant increase that would enable the changes to go forward. Armed with the Murphy report and the advice of the international consortium of EMS consultants, Murphy and the staff of the new Emergency Health Services Division of the Department of Health set to work implementing a province-wide, modern EMS network built around the three pillars of any valid health system- patient care, teaching and research.

To accomplish this within the mandate of the current Minister and government was no mean feat. There was no clean slate, no magic wands to wave. The very rumour of major changes set off speculation and insecurity among the providers of ambulance services and others, and the definitive and seemingly intransigent statements and actions of the Minister helped create an instability in the current ambulance service which, whatever its quality, it was the only one we had.[24] Although Bill 96, an 'Act to establish the Emergency Health Services Agency' was passed by the House in June of 1994, several years would go by before the government was able to engage a partner through a private-public agreement in 1997. This time period was required to reach agreements with over forty private providers within the province at the time, to transition into the new system and to begin upgrading of all personnel who would provide clinical care. The reform of the system over the first five years was intense and far-reaching. Each section of the Murphy Report required detailed planning in order to implement the recommendations that, for each element, were detailed and used as a benchmark to analyse the outcome after five years:

Ambulances/vehicles

Coupled with the variety of vehicles was the fact that government support for the ambulance operators up to that time for fleet renewal was, to say the least, spotty. The cost of replacing almost all the vehicles in the fleet immediately would have been staggering, but an innovative arrangement was proposed by the only ambulance manufacturing company in the Atlantic Region, Tri-Star Industries of Yarmouth.

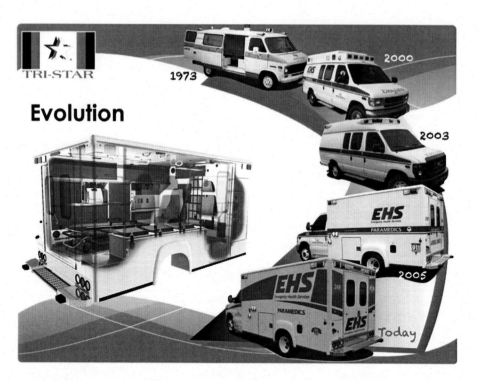

Figure 10.5 Tri-Star Industries was the Nova Scotia company contracted to completely refit the EHS system. They were already established in the international market.

Manufacturing ambulances and heavy specialised vehicles since 1973, Tri-Star Industries was active in some forty-five countries and was eager to be a part of the new system.(Figure 10.5) Through a leasing arrangement with EHS Nova Scotia and later with the care provider that employed the paramedics and delivered the clinical care in the system, modern designs were developed and total fleet renewal began immediately and progressed over the five years.

Although the vehicles would be owned by the Province, an improved leasing agreement allowed for a seamless fleet renewal system with regular improvements in vehicle and equipment as research and development by Tri-Star continue to respond to input from field personnel.

The original recommendations to the Minister included both ground and air ambulance service, with the medical directors of all programmes responsible to the Provincial EHS Medical Director. All vehicles would be staffed by two licenced paramedics unless a waiver was approved by the Medical Director, such as a Supervisor in the system or a special research of community paramedicine project. (Figure 10.6)

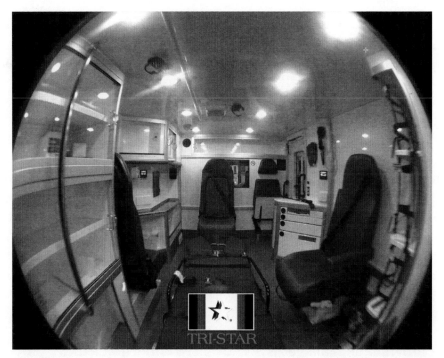

Figure 10.6 The interior design of the ground ambulances aimed at increasing the clinical space, ensuring room for more than one paramedic attendant and improving the safety of the internal environment.

Legislation

The legislation recommended by the Murphy Report clearly defined the corporate structure and the responsibilities of the EHS Division of the Ministry and the single private corporate structure delivering clinical care under the authority of the Provincial Medical Director. The contract with Emergency Medical Care, Inc. specified the role of both the regulator (EHS NS) and the contractor.

Organisation

Emergency Medical Services Nova Scotia (EHS NS) regulates the standards for the system as well as developing the clinical and billing policies. Personnel policies and scheduling are the responsibility of the contractor (Emergency Medical Care, Inc.); system performance measurements are based mostly on a system status management design.[25] It is noteworthy that the Provincial Medical Director is responsible directly to the Minister of Health and Wellness. He currently is ultimately responsible for all clinical guidelines for paramedic practice in Nova Scotia's EHS system. Field paramedics are guided in their duties initially by clinical judgement but expected to be wholly familiar with and adhere to the clinical guidelines developed over the twenty years of the service. A cadre of emergency physicians in all regions of the province is available for radio or cellphone consultation with all paramedics who are on duty throughout the system. (see below)

Programmes

Within the province-wide EHS network special programmes exist to support the primary clinical work of field paramedics both inside and outside the hospital. Paramedic practitioners who work in the tertiary Trauma and Emergency Centre are responsible to the emergency clinicians of the centre but are licenced as field paramedics under the recently-formed College of Paramedics of Nova Scotia.[26] Essential in the revamping of EHS in Nova Scotia was the creation of a regionalised Trauma Programme with a Medical Director responsible to the Provincial Medical Director. A full trauma registry is in place as well as a Provincial Advisory Board. The Trauma Programme Manager is an Advanced-care Paramedic.

Several initiatives already begun in the early nineties were continuing during this phase of EHS reform in the province, 1993-1997. Central to these was the need for the universal emergency number, 911, first initiated in 1959 in the city of Winnipeg as 999 after the British model.[27] The American Telephone and Telegraph Company (AT&T) announced in 1968 its intention to use the number 911 as the *'universal'* emergency contact number in the United States, but the process of implementation received little support such that at the end of 1972 only 17% of the population of the U.S. was covered by 911 service.[28] In order to avoid cross-border confusion, Winnipeg and the rest of Canada agreed to change from 999 to the 911 designation. Australia had adopted a national number "000" in 1961.[29] Nova Scotia followed suit with the 911 Act passing through the House in 1992, and completed in 1998, the first province-wide such service in Canada.[30]

Training

The initial years of instituting EHS reform were focused on two major essentials - clinical personnel and vehicles (ambulances). Both crucial elements of the system were in need of upgrading, in the case of many of the ambulance attendants by an expanded clinical and theoretical curriculum and in the case of vehicles by a standardised design and programme of replacement. The first challenge was taken up for several years by the creation of an EMT curriculum within the Allied Health School at the

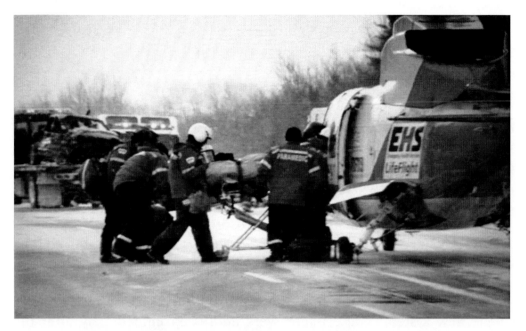

Figure 10.7 The Nova Scotia LifeFlight component provides helicopter or fixed-wing air transport. If needed, specialised teams: neonatal, obstetric, paediatric and others are available to supplement the paramedics.

Victoria General Hospital. All personnel had to complete the training before being licenced by EHS NS. Training modules were intensified so that the first class of paramedics graduated in 1999.[31] Since that time three nationally-accredited schools for primary and advanced Paramedic education have been established in all three Maritime provinces. Licencing and regulation in Nova Scotia has now been assumed by the College of Paramedics of Nova Scotia, as of April 1, 2017.[26] (Figure 10.7)

Tweaking the system

At the end of about five years during which the reformed system was fully functional, the Government of Nova Scotia commissioned a full report by an American team of consultants and gave them a mandate of examining every aspect of a modern EMS system and reporting on its performance to date, costs, value-for-dollar, and overall success in carrying out its duties to the citizens of the province. Even though the reformed system was in place for just over five years, the report card from the consultants issued in 2001 was unequivocal in its praise of the progress which had been made.

To quote the summary conclusions of the study group:

'The Nova Scotia EHS system has made dramatic improvements over the last few years. As performance continues to improve ... A pertinent question to be

asked is: Are the taxpayers of Nova Scotia receiving good value for the money spent on its emergency health services? The answer is an unequivocal-yes.' [32]

The path to the Academy

Establishing a modern emergency medical services system in which one of the main priorities is sustainability consists of more than providing funds and focusing mostly on ambulances and out-of-hospital care. A complete EMS system requires not only those basics but to take its proper place in the delivery of health care the system must be anchored to an academic teaching and research programme at all levels. Early in the reform process the elements that would provide this sustainability were mapped out and a strategy developed. The two main elements coming directly from the Murphy Report - ambulance fleet renewal and upgrading the training levels of current field personnel - were immediately tackled since ambulance service could not be interrupted to allow easier transition to the new system. These issues were addressed immediately after the contractual arrangements were complete. But the educational and research components, as expected, took longer.

Fortunately for the province, several physician leaders emerged with backgrounds in emergency medicine, beginning, as we have seen already, with Robert Scharf who assumed directorship of the Victoria General's Emergency Room in 1968 and laid down the beginnings of a modern Emergency Department. His ambulance training courses were integrated with the curriculum of the School of Allied Health at the Victoria General Hospital and after his sojourn at the L.A. County/USC Medical Center in the late seventies he returned to Dalhousie, eventually becoming the Director of the Emergency Department at the Saint John Regional Hospital in neighbouring New Brunswick.[13] From there he continued to press for the recognition of emergency medicine as a specialty within the Royal College, as he had in the seventies during his original tenure at Dalhousie.

Several other physicians arrived at the Victoria General who were key to the support of the EHS health system reform as they assumed leadership roles. By the early nineties at least five credentialed emergency physicians had taken up duties at Dalhousie, two of whom, Michael Murphy and Ian Morris had completed their emergency medicine residencies at the University of Colorado and returned to Dalhousie to finish training in anaesthesia as well. Dr. Ed Cain, a graduate of the University of Ottawa who became a Fellow of the Royal College in 1984, had been in place since the late seventies and went on to succeed Murphy as Director of EHS following creation of the Division within government. He played a decisive

162

role in the design of the clinical guidelines which govern paramedics' field practice and which were, and are, the most detailed evidence-based paramedic treatment protocols of any system.

With the creation of the specialty of Emergency Medicine by the Royal College of Physicians and Surgeons and the fellowship certification of the College of Family Physicians of Canada in 1980, it was considered essential to the development of the specialty within the province to establish a university programme that would provide for education in the specialty. Without this base there was concern by the framers of the design of EHS for Nova Scotia that the quality of paramedic training and clinical care would suffer. Certainly research, particularly with respect to outcome measurement as well as the formulation of clinical protocols, would be seriously impaired. The core of trained physicians committed to seeing this happen proved crucial to achieving these goals by the time the first phase of EHS reform was complete in the late nineties. Although the first submission for a residency to the required governing body failed to win approval, a second submission was successful following a more detailed description of the implications for this region of failing to achieve this essential component of clinical practice and specialty education. At the same time, the reformers within the Department of Health, including the Minister, were pressing to move forward with the creation of a specialty department within the Medical School, a fairly challenging move considering the constriction of the Health budget and plummeting federal transfer payments to both Health and Education.

Although the Emergency Department in the seventies was placed academically within the structure of the Department of Anaesthesia, the university had signaled late in the eighties that this needed to be revisited. On the retirement of Robert Scharf from Saint John and the Dalhousie Medical School, and with a growing cadre of young, articulate and committed emergency physicians in the main Emergency departments, the University approved the creation of an autonomous Department of Emergency Medicine under the Dean's office, the usual preliminary step to the creation of a fully sanctioned and independent Department within the Medical School structure. Chosen to head the new Department was Doug Sinclair, a young and talented clinician-administrator whose national influence and connections served the fledgling department well.[33] By 1998 the cycle was complete and the new specialty Department of Emergency Medicine took a seat around the table within the Faculty of Medicine.[34]

The way we are - 20 years on

Twenty years is but a brief span in the life of grand plans, but even so, at the end of five years the consultants of the Fitch Report would have to concede that Nova Scotia was at least holding its own and more than that, had made quite remarkable strides in providing high quality emergency health services to its citizens - and maybe even exceeded expectations. Few could deny the enormous challenge of providing emergency health services in a province with pockets of people separated by rugged coastline, the sea always close if not threatening, and weather changing almost from hour to hour. Many of these early challenges have been met, some are still dogging us; not a perfect picture, to be sure. But solid enough to hold on to and even build better for the next twenty years.

What, then, have been the major accomplishments that set this system apart from many others? What has changed? And where to from here?

System changes

One of the major problems in the early days of the evolution of mobile coronary care to what it is today, was the fact that the role and duties of emergency practitioners were not rigidly defined; in fact, many were through basic training before their roles were defined and it took even longer to give them legal status. In the sixties and seventies, in Miami, Eugene Nagel used telemetric/voice contact between physicians and paramedics not only to give a quasi-legal status to the extended role they assumed as physician extenders, but also to calm the distress of the less-than-enthusiastic fire chief who thought they were quite possibly playing hospital in the streets.[35] Mike Criley in Los Angeles had no solid legal protection for their programme or personnel for over a year until a California law, the Wedworth-Townsend Act was passed in 1970. Nurses rode on vehicles before the law defined what a paramedic could do, but voice/telemetry contact was required even after the Act was in force.[36] Most early EMS programmes in the United States required paramedic voice contact with an in-hospital nurse or physician in order to perform out-of-hospital duties. The design of the Nova Scotia system sought to avoid this, while ensuring all EHS team members - physicians, paramedics, communication/dispatching personnel - work closely with field paramedic teams and can, if requested, participate remotely in the total care of the patient or resolution of a situation.

This team concept starts with the Communications Centre's protocol system, the technology advancing over the twenty years such that

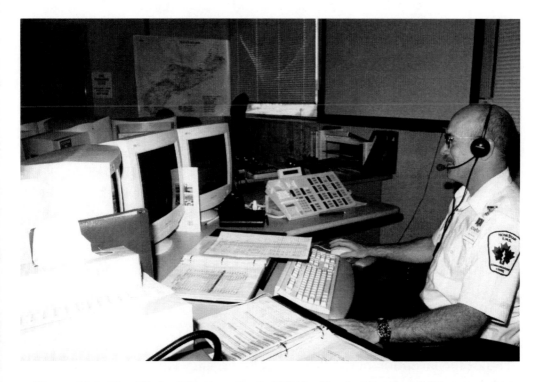

Figure 10.8 The Clinical Support Desk (CSD) offers back-up to field teams who may encounter clinical, legal or other issues. The experienced paramedic on duty has access to other consultants, directories of services, or information on medical and social programmes across the province.

determining location of call is now routine. Monitors track location and movement of all one hundred and fifty ambulances around the province, and computers record selected aspects of both vehicle and driver performance. Pre-arrival instructions were, and are, an inherent part of the Communications Centre's pivotal role. On-line emergency physicians are available on call for field team consultation at all times. This originally was done by means of an On-line Medical Control Physician (OLMCP) in each of the healthcare regions of the province responding to any field team voice calls from that area. This resulted in relatively minor or administrative calls to the EHS physicians for advice as to how the team should proceed in even non-urgent situations. That, in turn, led to an overload of the physician-paramedic consultation system with the risk inherent in having to stack calls. This has recently (2017) been replaced by establishing a central Clinical Support Desk (CSD) for round-the-clock peer-to-peer consultation in which both non-urgent clinical and administrative questions can be resolved safely and efficiently.(Figure 10.8) Advanced care paramedics staff the CSD and have access to computerised detailed information connecting government ministries, social service agencies, health related community resources and law enforcement. In addition, direct communication can be established by the CSD between the on-line EHS Physician and the field medics, or all three parties may be connected.

It is important to note that these CSD-practitioners are not providing orders to paramedics in the field (as this would be a function reserved for online EMS physicians) but act as a resource to their frontline colleagues as they have more reference material at their disposal than a paramedic crew in a patient's living room or in an ambulance on the side of a highway. Field teams report there is great value in discussing the care plan with a colleague removed from the situation as this can mitigate cognitive biases that may be at play when making clinical decisions. Recently the CSD programme has expanded to handle many mandatory calls that were traditionally fielded by the on-line physicians. This occurred, not coincidentally, around the same time (April 1, 2017) that paramedics became a self regulated health profession in Nova Scotia.

Field practice

Since the inception of the Provincial Emergency Health Services system, paramedics have operated under liberal protocols (compared to almost all North American EMS systems) and they have the benefit of significant autonomy in clinical decision making. These prospective protocols, recently replaced by Clinical Practice Guidelines (CPGs),[37] are based on high-quality evidence informed by the Prehospital Evidence Based Practice Project of the Dalhousie University Department of Emergency Medicine, Division of EMS - the largest pre-hospital evidence based medicine repository of its kind.[38] Along with these CPGs, there is, and has always been, round-the-clock online medical consultation available for paramedics on complex cases or when requiring a mandatory physician consult for orders if indicated in the CPG. CPGs requiring physician contact are few and typically are required for high-risk, low-volume interventions or presentations such as tranexamic acid (TXN) administration in severe blood loss in non-trauma patients, post-partum haemorrhage, etc. In addition, most field teams would favour online physician consultation in cases of high-risk 'non transport' in which the safety of not transporting the patient, according to recent evidence, is ambiguous. The ability to discuss non-urgent issues with the CSD rather than every time with the EHS on-line physician has reduced physician overload considerably. Contact with the on-line physician before applying a clinical protocol is left to the discretion of the field team, unless such contact may be obligatory under the guidelines.

166

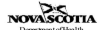
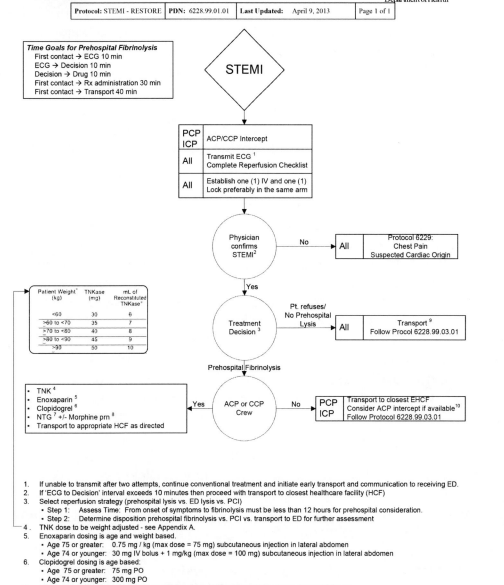

1. If unable to transmit after two attempts, continue conventional treatment and initiate early transport and communication to receiving ED.
2. If 'ECG to Decision' interval exceeds 10 minutes then proceed with transport to closest healthcare facility (HCF)
3. Select reperfusion strategy (prehospital lysis vs. ED lysis vs. PCI)
   - Step 1: Assess Time: From onset of symptoms to fibrinolysis must be less than 12 hours for prehospital consideration.
   - Step 2: Determine disposition prehospital fibrinolysis vs. PCI vs. transport to ED for further assessment
4. TNK dose to be weight adjusted - see Appendix A.
5. Enoxaparin dosing is age and weight based.
   - Age 75 or greater: 0.75 mg / kg (max dose = 75 mg) subcutaneous injection in lateral abdomen
   - Age 74 or younger: 30 mg IV bolus + 1 mg/kg (max dose = 100 mg) subcutaneous injection in lateral abdomen
6. Clopidogrel dosing is age based:
   - Age 75 or greater: 75 mg PO
   - Age 74 or younger: 300 mg PO
7. NTG - up to 3 doses only and if patient remains stable (SBP > 90 and HR between 50 and 100 bpm).
8. Be cautious with Morphine dosing (2.5 mg increments)
9. Transport to closest HCF capable of ED Lysis, or destination directed by ED physician; notify ED of ETA; print 'STEMI Decision' ECG for handover to ED
10. Consider ACP intercept if intercept is faster than closest ED arrival.

Figure 10.9 Application of each Clinical Guideline is based on the clinical judgement of the paramedic in consultation, as needed, with the on-duty Online Medical Control Physician. In the event that ST-segment elevation is detected the clinical intervention is determined by travel time to the PCI unit in consultation with that team.

One of the first Clinical Guidelines developed in the revised system of protocols and requirements for online physician consult was the field intervention in suspected myocardial infarction with ST-segment elevation, or STEMI. In truth, field practice has come full circle since 1966 when the first 'Flying Squad' rolled out from the Royal Victoria Hospital grounds to the first case of myocardial infarction. Belfast early on suggested that, although the phrase wasn't used then, *'tissue **was** time, and time **was** tissue.'* The difference in the 21st century is that we can now do much more to attack the main cause of the problem - the clot- after the initial management of pain and dysrhythmias. This protocol relies on the expeditious application of interventions that have stood the test of time, including thrombolysis for cases in which a time delay would occur due to geography, weather, traffic patterns, etc. This guideline requires a coordinated effort of the field paramedic team with the PCI (Percutaneous Coronary Intervention) team and the EMS physician on duty at the tertiary care Department of Emergency Medicine (Queen Elizabeth II Health Sciences Centre, Halifax). (Figure 10.9) The PCI unit can provide definitive reperfusion procedures such as stent placement. Field thrombolysis by the paramedic field team is applied in a carefully constructed guideline if transport to the PCI Team is delayed by distance or by weather. Both air transport and ground critical care transport can be used to retrieve STEMI patients from distances beyond sixty or ninety minutes from Halifax. In these cases in which time is of the essence, the outcome will depend largely on the collaborative effort of both field and in-hospital teams working together using the facilities of PCI or, in cases more remote from the facility, the judicious use of tenecteplase (TNK) when indicated by paramedic field teams.

It should be noted that all clinical guidelines are the result of ongoing discussion, debate and deliberation among staff paramedics and physicians from the Department of Emergency Medicine and Division of EMS of Dalhousie Medical School. Protocols are reviewed and updated continually, the foundation for these reviews being the Canadian Pre-hospital Evidence-based Practice (PEP) project based in the Department. The PEP project is a collaborative effort of Canada's EMS Physicians, paramedics, Dalhousie University Division of EMS and Emergency Health Services Nova Scotia.[38] The website is monitored and monthly reports generated of the traffic logging on to the website, including the origin of these world-wide contacts.

Research

The Division of EMS of the Department of Emergency Medicine at Dalhousie is responsible for generating projects emanating from the Department of Emergency Medicine or any project in which EHS collaborates. There is close cooperation in these endeavours with EMC,Inc (Medavie Health Services), the contracted agency for EHS services in Nova Scotia, as well as with Emergency Health Services of the Department of Health and Wellness of the government of Nova Scotia. Research projects are generated from the work of paramedics, particularly those working full-time on projects affiliated with the Division,[39,40] but a significant surge of papers and projects has resulted recently from the Research-in-Medicine project of the Faculty of Medicine. This programme requires all undergraduate medical students to develop, carry out and report on a four-year research project under a preceptor from any Department within the faculty. A major source of projects is through residents of the department, with departmental faculty members supervising, or they may be generated by Faculty members themselves.

Research continues to be a major contributor to the life and health of the department at the medical school, and the Division of Emergency Medical Services has helped greatly to make it equally important to the EHS system in the province. There are significant advantages to the cross-appointments which the Division and members of the Faculty enjoy with EHS Nova Scotia, an arm of the ministry, and EMCI (Medavie Health Services), the provider of ground and air service. Data collection is more efficient, priorities are more readily set and monitored and there is a certain economy of scale, rather than a duplication of effort or budgetary allotments. This appears to be unique in jurisdiction-wide service-oriented systems in which silos and protected turf can often impede the progress of any initiative, whether inside or outside a hospital setting. The advantage of smaller size also shows itself. The province is small enough to provide a system in which most players in the health field know each other and therefore tend to cooperate. However, there is a sufficient number of patients to provide data for most studies, or at least a detection of trends, with perhaps the exception of certain types of trauma, particularly penetrating wounds.

Changing and expanding roles

Early on in the planning of the EHS system for Nova Scotia it was realised that, given the rural and sometimes remote nature of much of the province it would be necessary to enlist as many citizens and organisations as possible in a modern emergency health services system. There were active and valuable resources already in place. The Heart and Stroke Foundation, along with its excellent programmes aimed at prevention and other aspects of cardiovascular disease were supportive of citizen training in CPR, as were St. John's Ambulance, the Canadian Red Cross and the Canadian Life-saving Society, all well known for their training programmes for citizens in first-aid and water safety. Fire services within the province, most of which operated as community endeavours staffed by volunteers, played a primary role in EHS as a part of the wider effort specialising in extrication techniques and rescue, CPR and initial management of the emergency, particularly the use of Automated External Defibrillators (AED's) following immediate application of basic CPR techniques.[41] The 'First Responder Programme' was initiated and is now an integral part of EHS Nova Scotia, reporting directly to the EHS Provincial Medical Director.[42] Although most 'Medical First Responders' (MFR) are associated with Fire Services in the province, others groups - life-guards, police/ RCMP and security personnel - are part of the wider programme.

In the early development of the EHS system for Nova Scotia, the consultants were asked to imagine the 'paramedic' to be a generic term with no real restrictions - geographic, academic, or sociological, and to create a role in the health system which would be defined by perceived needs in patient care or gaps which need to be filled. This thinking gave rise to some anxiety on the part of those taking part in the discussion, but much good came of it. Rather than define the role geographically- as a health care giver who works outside of hospital in an ambulance - the exercise looked at what might be needed to deliver episodic and emergency care and to serve as a conduit through the often confusing maze called a health care system. At least in the discussion we came away feeling that this newly arrived health care professional could not be readily defined and that the system be developed to fill these perceived gaps rather than define the paramedic. Flexibility would be the key. In essence, given the nature of episodic round-the-clock care, most felt it was likely that paramedics could fill gaps and expand their role in primary care delivery.

The subject of training and educational levels was left unspecified, at least looking farther down the road. This discussion led then to the definition not only of roles but also of the necessity of a career ladder for the paramedic in a progressive system. Over the twenty or so years since the initial discussion took place, EHS paramedics in Nova Scotia have assumed roles that go well beyond the traditional concept of the ambulance driver. Innovation has led to a gradual but definite expansion of their role within the health system, somewhat a result of initial planning, but more so occurring because of the gaps that became obvious in the traditional approach to primary care delivery. A major factor in the relatively rapid expansion of the role of EHS personnel in the health care system was the quality of performance of paramedic crews in their traditional role as responders to medical crises and the rapid growth of public trust in the maturing profession.

Thinking outside the box

It is clear that the introduction of a regionalised emergency health service for the province offered even to rural and remote regions the likelihood that health care services would be improved through standardised personnel training, equipment and clinical protocols. The trend towards grouping specialised care into larger centres as well as the apparent decline in the numbers of health care personnel locating in rural areas presented a dilemma for public health and primary care delivery. Added to this was the fact that EHS personnel posted to small stations in remote areas could experience significant skill decay without at least occasional exposure to medical emergencies.[43] Perhaps the most challenging expansion of emergency services had been scheduled in the first years of the regionalised programme was on the islands of Briar and Long Island, located off the southwest coast of Nova Scotia at the entrance to the Bay of Fundy. The nearest community hospital was located at Digby on the mainland, approximately one hundred kilometres from the two ferries that transported travelers first to Long and then to Briar Island. An innovative programme fielded a health team led by the two paramedic units, one on each island, with a mainland-based Nurse Practitioner who visited the Island, the local regional EMS director and the Digby hospital. The results of an in-depth study showed how community health services were improved, transportation costs for citizens lowered, new programmes were introduced and visits to the emergency department, as well as admissions to the Digby hospital were reduced significantly. Unexpected improvements in chronic health disease parameters were seen over the five years of the study, and citizen satisfaction was uniformly high.[44] The success of this pilot lead to the formation by the Department of Health and Wellness of a network of rural **Collaborative Emergency Centres** in selected communities in the northern and eastern regions of the province which have been recognised by a national accrediting body as significant examples of innovation in health care delivery.[45] (Figure 10.10)

Nova Scotia has the third-highest percentage of citizens over the age of sixty-five in Canada, at about 14% of the population. Early on in the development of EHS within the province, it was realised that these older

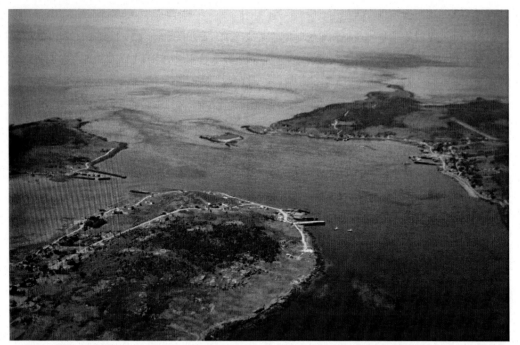

Figure 10.10 Briar and Long Island are two islands which challenged the system of providing rural primary and emergency care in the province. Located at the end of a long neck of land along the Bay of Fundy, Briar Island is reached by ferry after crossing to Long Island from Digby neck in the mainland. An innovative and collaborative programme was designed to provide for the care of the people of the islands, with quite remarkable success.

citizens often had to rely on the emergency health service not only for conditions requiring immediate intervention but also for less medically urgent, but still important problems they faced. Frequently those problems would lead them to busy emergency departments in which they might be forced to wait, often uncomfortably in unfamiliar surroundings and with few options. Faced with this growing problem, EHS planners and field teams initiated a pilot project, The **Extended Care Paramedic Programme** in which advanced-trained paramedics attended residents of long-term care facilities and, when appropriate, treatment was done within the facility along with the expediting of radiological or other testing in hospital if required. The result of the project was that transports from nursing homes to emergency departments in the Central Region were reduced by almost 50% and with call-backs resulting in emergency department admission less than 3%.[46] Both patient and staff satisfaction with the programme was high, and this innovation in the system won national recognition after the results were published following peer review.[47]

The success of the Briar-Long Island collaborative care project combined with the national recognition of the extended-care innovation plan served as the basis for the **Special Patient Programme** (SPP) of EHS. Before this programme, patients in palliative care or who had special needs requiring medical advice or intervention would have to be taken to an emergency department if 911 had been called. Under this plan, home-care patients who have special needs, particularly those in palliative care, are registered in the data base which will identify them when a Paramedic team is requested through the EHS Communications Centre via 911. Patients with rare conditions, unique needs or those with special medical equipment or apparatus can also be included in the registry. When the ground ambulance is dispatched by the Communications Centre, the paramedic crew is notified and its computer can provide information on the special needs that should be met during the call, including whether the ambulance response should be 'silent' (that is, without warning lights and siren) or if it is urgent.[48] On arrival and after assessing the problem, the paramedic crew can seek further information or advice by means of the Clinical Support Desk officer or by direct consultation with the Online Medical Oversight Physician (OLMOP). In most cases the problems can be addressed in the home or institution in consultation with the wishes of the patient and the family so that comfort care plans and patients' decisions take priority. Often, both patients enrolled in the programme and family members comment on the greater sense of security this brings, knowing they are but a phone call away from advice and help that can be provided quickly, quietly and without fuss, twenty-four hours a day.

Initially, as plans were being made to introduce the elements of the revised system in 1994, a recurrent theme in the discussions was the issue of the career path that might eventually be created for what the Minister believed was a legitimate profession. He was reminded of the dilemma of military 'corpsmen', or paramedics as they were eventually called, who, on discharge from the services in both the Korean and Vietnam conflicts, and others, hit a professional brick wall in the United States [49]. They found themselves unable to practice their very considerable clinical skills because there was no job description for them, and seldom any reciprocal academic credits. Many, as a result, went into public safety careers - police, fire, private security - or became orderlies in hospitals, and some went on to medicine or on to nursing school. But none of these vocations allowed them to practice the skills, clinical and otherwise, that they had been trained so well to do. It was felt by several consultants and the Minister that the Nova Scotia system could avoid that loss of clinical skills as the workforce became older and much more experienced by providing another rung on the career ladder for paramedics to reach if they wished to achieve an expanded role in the health system. The eventual model would be designed to ensure that there would be a seamless connection between care in a field setting (i.e. paramedic care) and the more comprehensive emergency care and management which might be provided by a paramedic working with physicians in emergency hospitals and trauma centres as Practitioners. This was achieved, with significant outcomes, with the programme of Emergency Department paramedics now working in the tertiary Trauma and Emergency Centre of the province. There is growing evidence that the next step must be to expand such programmes.[50,51]

Where we were, where we are and where we want to be

The most recent development in the story that is EHS Nova Scotia and an achievement which should be celebrated is the inauguration of the **College of Paramedics of Nova Scotia**, the acknowledgment by the citizens of the province through their legislative representatives that a new health profession has sprung from the work of the last twenty years and built on the foundation put in place years before. The College assumes the credentialing, licencing, regulation and discipline of all paramedics within the EHS system of the province.[52]

The past twenty years has seen the development of an infrastructure in Emergency Health Services in Nova Scotia which is now mature enough to withstand further reform - designed around the fact that we have been, and are, an almost perfect laboratory for evaluation and research into the clinical interventions and organisational structure of a centralised system. As in all of health care, change is not only inevitable, it is desirable.

The successes, and the adjustments of the not-quite successes, drive the system to greater efforts to ensure the quality of the care delivered and that the citizen - the patient - must always be the central focus of what we do. Despite the important details of every single protocol, covering every need and eventuality, the strength of any health system lies in how the practitioner imparts a sense of caring, confidence and competence. In the small world of Nova Scotia, a benchmark was set and for the most part, all things being human, it was reached. Just as, in 1967, the spark that lit up a part of our world came out of Belfast we have tried to build on that spirit of innovation and measured daring, have gone perhaps beyond Belfast, and we trust the citizens within our sea-bound coast will agree we're all the better for it.

References

1. Santy P, Moulinier M, Marquis D. Le choc traumatique dans les blessures de guerre, analyse d'observations – Bull Med Soc Chir 1918;44:205.
2. Neel S. Army aeromedical evacuation procedures in Vietnam: implications for rural America. JAMA 1968;204:99-103.
3. Kelman HR, Lane DS. Use of the hospital emergency room in relation to use of private physicians. Am J Pub Health 1976; 66:1189-91.
4. Merritt AK. The rise of emergency medicine in the sixties: paving a new entrance to the house of medicine. J Hist Med Allied Sci 2014;69:251-93.
5. Farrington JD. Death in a ditch. Bull Am Coll Surg 1967; 52:121-30.
6. Safar P, Brose RA. Ambulance design and equipment for resuscitation. Arch Surg 1965;90:343-8.
7. Whitehead J. Paying for health care - the top five things you need to know. Nova Scotia Health Authority. Halifax, NS. Nov 15, 2011. Accessed June 28, 2017. Available from: [http://www.cdha.nshealth.ca/media-centre/2011-11/paying-health-care-top-five-things-you-need-know]
8. Pantridge JF, Geddes JS. A mobile intensive-care unit in the management of myocardial infarction. Lancet 1967;2:271-3.
9. Government of Canada. Canada's health care system. Available from:https://www.canada.ca/en/health-canada/services/canada-health-care-system.html [Accessed 20th June 2017].
10. Committee on Trauma, Shock and Anesthesia. Accidental Death and Disability: the Neglected Disease of Modern Society. Washington DC: National Academy of Sciences-National Research Council; Sept,1966.
11. Ambulance Operators Association of Nova Scotia [Internet]. [Place unknown]. [Cited 2017Jul 8]. Available from: https://www.revolvy.com/main/index.php?s=Ambulance%20Operators%20Association%20of%20Nova%20Scotia
12. McAlister C, Twohig P. The Check-off: a precursor of medicare in Canada? CMAJ 2005;173:1504-6.
13. Obituary. Robert F. Scharf. CMAJ 2007;177:987.
14. Stewart RD. Interview by Brian Zink, Boularderie Island, Nova Scotia, 2004; quoted in Zink BJ. Anyone, anything, anytime: a history of emergency medicine. Philadelphia: Mosby; 2006. p 151.
15. Lewis AJ, Ailshie G, Criley JM: Pre-hospital cardiac care in a paramedical mobile intensive care unit. Calif Med 1972;117:1-8.

16. Zink BJ. Anyone, anything, anytime: a history of emergency medicine. Philadelphia: Mosby; 2006. p 202-3.

17. Gesztes A, Mezei A. Topical anesthesia of the skin by liposome-encapsulated tetracaine. Anesth Analg 1988;67:1079-81.

18. Hung OR, Stewart RD. Lightwand intubation: I. A new intubating device. Can J Anaesth1995;42:820-5.

19. Hung OR,Whynot SC,Varvel JR, Shafer SL,Mezei M. Pharmacokinetics of inhaled liposome-encapsulated fentanyl. Anesthesiology. 1995;83:277-84

20. Hung OR, Stewart RD. Remembering the famous and forgotten in medicine. Anesth Analges 2014;119:1005-6.

21. MacLeod JJ. Health care reform in Nova Scotia: a study in pressure-group politics 1993-1996. Unpublished thesis Masters. Wolfville: Acadia University; 1996.

22. Murphy MF, Petley-Jones A. Report: Emergency Health Services in Nova Scotia. Halifax: Department of Health; 1994.

23. Fire Services Senior Officials Committee. An assessment of selected past reports regarding the efficiency and effectiveness of Nova Scotia emergency services. Halifax: Fire Services Senior Officials Committee; 2012 p. 19-24. Available from: http://novascotia.ca/news/docs/2015/06/01/Fire-Services-Report-ANNEX-B-Literature-Review.pdf

24. MacLeod JJ. Health care reform in Nova Scotia: a study in pressure-group politics 1993-1996. Unpublished thesis Masters. Wolfville: Acadia University; 1996. p 84-90.

25. Dean S. The origins of system status management. Emerg Med Serv 2004;33:116-8.

26. An Act Respecting the Practice of Paramedicine [Online]. [http://nslegislature.ca/legc/bills/62nd_2nd/1st_read/b123.htm]. 2017 [cited 2017 Jul 13]. Available from: Office of the Legislative Council, Nova Scotia House of Assembly.

27. CBC Digital Archives. [Online] [cited 2017 Jul 14]; Available from: URL: http://www.cbc.ca/archives/entry/winnipeggers-call-999-for-help

28. NENA The 911 Association. 911 Origin and history. [Online]. [cited 2017 Jul 14]; Available from: URL:https://www.nena.org/?page=911overviewfacts

29. Triple Zero (000). [Online] 2011 [cited 2017Jul14]; Available from: URL: https://www.triplezero.gov.au/Pages/default.aspx

30. Government of Nova Scotia. 911 Fact Sheet. [Online]. 2012 [cited 2017 Jul 15]; Available from:https://novascotia.ca/dma/emo/

resources/docs/911_Fact_Sheet_Sept_2012.pdf

31. First class of advanced level paramedics graduates. 1999. Available from: URL: https://novascotia.ca/news/release/?id=19990623006

32. Fitch and Associates, LLC. Performance evaluation of Nova Scotia emergency health services. Platte City, MO: Nova Scotia Department of Health. [cited 2001 Nov]. Available from: [https://novascotia.ca/dhw/publications/Performance_Evaluation_EHS%20.pdf].

33. MacLeod JJ. Health care reform in Nova Scotia: a study in pressure-group politics 1993-1996. Unpublished thesis Masters. Wolfville: Acadia University; 1996. p 96.

34. Editorial. Royal College recognizes emergency medicine as primary specialty. CMAJ 1981;124:1357.

35. Nagel EL, Hirschman JC, Mayer PW, Dennis F. Telemetry of physiological data: an aid to fire-rescue personnel in a metropolitan area. Southern Med J 1968;61:598-601.

36. Lewis AJ, Ailshie G, Criley JM. Pre-hospital cardiac care in a paramedical mobile intensive care unit. Calif Med 1972;117:1-8.

37. Emergency Health Services EHS ground ambulance clinical program documents. [Online]. 2013 [cited 2017 Jul 17]; Available from: URL:https://novascotia.ca/dhw/ehs/clinical-program-documents.asp

38. Canadian prehospital evidence-based practice (PEP). [Online]. 2012 [cited 2017 Jul 17]; Available from : URL: https://emspep.cdha.nshealth.ca/Introduction.aspx

39. Jensen JL, Petrie DA, Cain E, Travers AH. The Canadian prehospital evidence-based protocols project: knowledge translation in emergency medical services care. Acad Emerg Med 2009;16:668-73.

40. Goldstein JP, Andrew MK, Travers A. Frailty in older adults using pre-hospital care and the emergency department: a narrative review. Can Geriatrics J 2012;15:16-22.

41. Sanna T, La Torre G, de Waure C, Scapigliati A, Ricciardi W, Dello Russo A et al. Cardiopulmonary resuscitation alone vs. cardiopulmonary resuscitation plus automated external defibrillator use by non-healthcare professionals: a meta-analysis on 1583 cases of out-of-hospital cardiac arrest. Resuscitation 2008;76:226-31.

42. Nova Scotia Medical First Responder Program Emergency Health Services. [Online]. 2012 [cited 2017 Jul 16]; Available from: URL: http://www.ehsmfr.ca/Pages/Program-Overview.aspx

43. Gold LS, Eisenberg MS. The effect of paramedic experience on survival from cardiac arrest. Prehosp Emerg Care 2009;13:341-4.

44. Martin-Misener R, Downe-Wamboldt B, Cain E, Girouard M. Cost

effectiveness and outcomes of a nurse-practitioner-paramedic-family physician model of care: the Long and Brier Islands study. Prim Health Care Res 2009;10:14-25.

45. Accreditation Canada. Collaborative Emergency Centres (CEC's). [Online]. 2013 [cited 2017 Jul 16]; Available from: URL:https://accreditation.ca/collaborative-emergency-centres-cecs

46. Jensen JL, Marshall EG, Carter AJE, Boudreau M, Bure F, Travers AH. Impact of a novel collaborative long-term care-EMS model: a before-and-after cohort analysis of an extended-care paramedic program. Prehosp Emerg Care 2016;20:111-16.

47. Paramedic program reducing emergency room congestion. CMAJ 2011 12;183:E631-2.

48. Nova Scotia Department of Health and Wellness. Special patient program: information for health care professionals. [Online]. 2016 [cited 2017 Jul 17]; Available from: URL:https://novascotia.ca/dhw/palliativecare/documents/SPP_Health_Care_Professionals.PDF

49. Former medics find themselves on bottom rung in civilian field. [Online]. 2017 [cited 2017 Jul 14]; Available from: URL:https://www.stripes.com/news/veterans/former-medics-find-themselves-on-bottom-rung-in-civilian-field-1.344392#.WWuK64QrL3g

50. Campbell S, Petrie D, MacKinley R, Froese P, Etsell P, Warren DA et al. Procedural sedation and analgesia facilitator – expanded scope role for paramedics in the emergency department. J Emerg Prim Health Care 2008;6:1-12.

51. Campbell SG, Janes SE, MacKinley RP, Froese PC, Harris S, Etsell GR et al. Patient management in the emergency department by advanced care paramedics. Healthcare Manage Forum 2012;25:26-31.

52. Nova Scotia College of Paramedics. About the College. [Online] 2017 [Cited Jul 18]; Available from: URL: https://www.cpns.ca/

Chapter 11

Biography of Frank Pantridge

Frank Pantridge was born in Hillsborough, County Down, Northern Ireland on 3rd October 1916. At that time only a few hundred people lived in the village of Hillsborough, which was about twenty kilometres from Belfast. His parents were small landowners with a farm on the Ballygowan Road just outside the village. Frank was the oldest of three children with a younger brother (Herbert) and sister (Emily). Their father died in 1927 when Frank was eleven years old; his mother lived to her ninetieth year. (Figure 11.1).

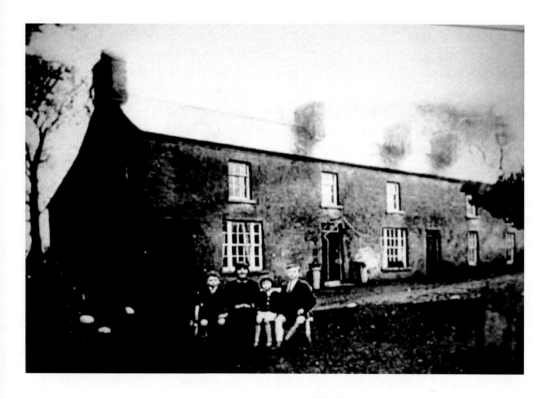

Figure 11.1 The Pantridge house, Hillsborough, circa 1926.
Left to right: Herbert, Mrs Pantridge, Emily, Frank.

179

His early education was at the local Downshire School in the village. For high school he took the bus to the Friends' School in Lisburn – a market town some eight kilometres from Hillsborough. Pantridge recounted some details of his early education in his autobiography, *An Unquiet Life*. By his own admission his academic school performance was *'less than average'*. He was not athletically inclined and throughout his life showed moderate disdain for those who were. His only sporting endeavour was to play cricket for the Hillsborough village team, where he *'had a modest reputation as a slip fielder'*; a position that requires very fast reflexes. He later indulged in salmon fishing and played an occasional low grade but determined game of golf.

The sons of landowners were often directed into one of the three professions – the church, law or medicine. As he wrote *'I was certainly not the clerical type and from an early age I had shown scant respect for the law so I was directed into medicine.'* He admired the local, highly respected, general practitioner and declared, *'My ambition was to become a village doctor somewhere in Northern Ireland.'* Thus, in the autumn of 1934 he entered the Queen's University of Belfast to begin the five-year course in medicine. In his second year he contracted diphtheria, complicated by heart block. He managed to catch up the time lost and pass a supplementary exam after appealing his case to the Dean, who overruled the unsympathetic Botany professor's insistence that he repeat the year. In his final clinical examination in medicine he was given the case of a boy with a solid left chest. Pantridge diagnosed this as a pleural effusion but the examiner, a consultant chest physician, said he was wrong and the patient had pneumonia. Failure in this major medical case would have meant that he would fail the entire examination. Pantridge was convinced he was right and persuaded the house officer on the ward to perform a pleural tap on the patient and took the confirmatory fluid to the home of the Professor of Medicine, Sir William Thomson. He handed the specimen to the maid at the door along with a note outlining the situation. He passed with honours. An early manifestation of his strong sense of self-belief, distrust of authority and tenacity that would become the hallmark of his character and help him survive the hardship ahead. Pantridge claimed, *'I had an undistinguished undergraduate career. I was lucky to graduate.'* However, the fact that he graduated with honours, a feat only achieved by less than ten percent of the class belies this modest assertion – notwithstanding his coup with the pleural effusion.

On 1st August 1939 Frank Pantridge started his houseman's year (internship) as a resident medical physician at the Royal Victoria Hospital

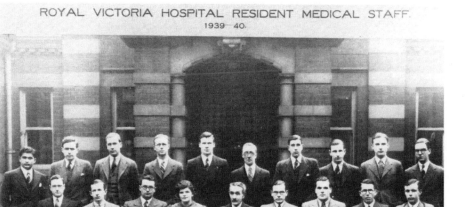

Figure 11.2
Royal Victoria Hospital, Resident Medical Staff, 1939-40. JFP seated on far right.

(RVH), Belfast. (Figure 11.2). Pantridge heard Chamberlain's declaration of war on Sunday 3rd September, 1939 and the following day he and eleven of the thirteen house officers in the RVH volunteered at the local recruiting office. Ever since the Belfast Medical School opened in 1835 there had been a strong tradition of doctors from Northern Ireland serving in the British colonial and armed services – in part due to the overproduction of medical graduates. For example, of those qualifying in the years 1919-1934, 85% left the province to find employment.

Pantridge had grown up in the aftermath of World War I: *'At the Downshire School in Hillsborough in the early twenties, much of the talk amongst the youngsters concerned the Battle of the Somme and the local citizens who had been killed there.'* He was aware that in the battle on 1st July 1916 the Ulster Division took more than 5,000 casualties and four soldiers were awarded the highest medal for valour – the Victoria Cross.

Pantridge and his volunteer colleagues remained in the RVH to gain more experience until their call-up in April 1940. During his early army training in Headingly, Yorkshire he was drafted to take part in a mission to occupied Norway. However, due to his lack of skiing experience he was

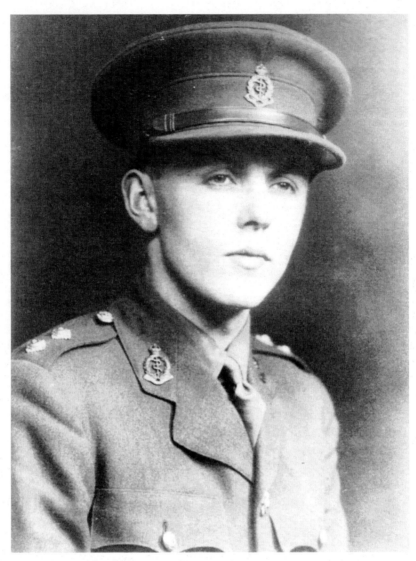

Figure 11.3 Lieutenant Frank Pantridge 1939.

removed from the group – none of whom survived. After basic training in England, he was posted to Singapore and there seconded to the Second Battalion Gordon Highlanders. (Figure 11.3). He found the military routine 'boring' and frequently questioned the logic of his superior officers. On one occasion he narrowly escaped court-martial when he had the temerity to talk back to a regular army Colonel who chastised him for reducing a man's dislocated shoulder, rather than following protocol and referring the case to a surgeon.

The dull military routine was shattered in January 1942 when the Japanese invaded Malaya, culminating in the surrender of Singapore on 15th February 1942. In the final days of the battle for Singapore Pantridge was awarded the Military Cross (MC) for bravery in the field. This high honour was rarely given to doctors and not often awarded in a losing campaign.

The citation to support the award read: *"During the operations in Johore and Singapore.....as medical officer attached to the 2/Gordons, this officer worked unceasingly under the most adverse conditions of continuous bombing and shelling and was an inspiring example to all with whom he came into contact. He was absolutely cool under the heaviest fire and completely regardless of his own personal safety at all times."*

As a prisoner of war he remained medical officer to the ill-fated 'F' force of some 7000 Australian and British soldiers in the slave labour camps building the Siam-Burma railway – subsequently made famous in the film, *Bridge over the River Kwai*. Pantridge developed severe beriberi and, too ill to carry out his duties, was transferred to the infamous Tanbaya 'death camp' on the Siam-Burma border. He was one of the few to survive the camp; *'I will not leave my bloody bones in Burma.'* The stubborn combative nature of Frank Pantridge's character was well known to his friends. One of whom, upon learning of his capture at Singapore said, *'God help the bloody Japanese'*; this was before their unspeakable cruelty toward their captives was known.

By the end of 1943 the few survivors who had built the railway were returned to the Changi jail in Singapore – only 125 of the original 7000 were fit for work duties. The Japanese capitulated in August 1945 and Pantridge was liberated on 11th September when a hospital ship arrived in Singapore. As it happened the ship's medical officer, Tom Milliken, was a former classmate and he described their meeting as follows:
"I found Pantridge in one of the many huts. He was trying to get on a shirt but with little success because of the weakened and wasted arms.....The upper half of his body was emaciated, skin and bones. The lower half was bloated with the dropsy of beri-beri. The most striking thing was the blue eyes that blazed with defiance. He was a physical wreck but his spirit was obviously unbroken. The eyes said it was indestructible....." He weighed under 70lb (32kg).

Pantridge remained critical of the politicians and higher military authorities in England who left Singapore without naval or air support and contributed to the fall of the island; history has substantiated his opinion. He witnessed the extreme cruelty and brutality of the Japanese and never forgave them.

With relief he returned to Ulster, *'I breathed the free air of County*

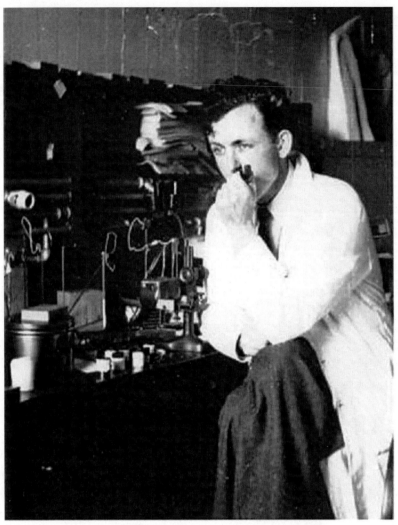

Figure 11.4 JFP in Ann Arbor, Michigan 1948.

Down, God's own country.' After completing the remaining six months of his houseman's year he found no vacancies in general practice. The only position available was a supernumerary lectureship in pathology. He took this and completed a project on the effect of beriberi on the pig heart – the conducting system of which is similar to the human. In 1946 he completed the examination for the higher degree of MD and in 1947 passed, at his first attempt, the examination for membership of the College of Physicians of London (MRCP)– which had a failure rate of more than 90%. In 1948 he was awarded a scholarship to study at the University of Michigan in Ann Arbor with Frank Wilson, at that time the world's authority on electrocardiography (Figure 11.4). There he acquired a good knowledge of electronics, which was invaluable when he later became involved with the development of defibrillators.

Returning to Belfast in 1949 he became registrar (resident) to the medical unit of Sir William Thomson. In 1951 Pantridge was appointed consultant physician to the outpatient medical department of the RVH with six beds in Wards 5 and 6. Two years later he became Physician in charge of the Cardiac Unit which comprised Wards 5 and 6. Although designated for patients with heart disease, twice a week the wards had to accept the general emergency medical admissions that came through the Casualty Department. In total there were almost fifty beds in the two wards – Ward 5 female and Ward 6 male.

Upon his appointment as consultant in 1951 Pantridge turned his attention to a very common problem at that time, rheumatic heart disease. In particular, the complication of mitral stenosis caused the death of many sufferers in their mid to late-thirties. Before he left the United States in 1949 Pantridge visited Philadelphia and saw Charles Bailey carry out mitral valvotomy and was impressed with the results. By 1951 he had convinced the thoracic surgeons in Belfast to start the procedure. Between 1951 and 1976 some 2500 patients had the operation performed in the RVH at the hands of three thoracic surgeons: John Bingham, Tom Smiley and Morris Stevenson. Pantridge conducted the whole performance: selection of patients for surgery, preoperative preparation and postoperative care. Only the operation was carried out in the surgical theatre, with Pantridge present, '..... *striding up and down the room and offering irritatingly astute advice at all times'*, as one anaesthetist put it. Immediately after the operation the patient was transferred back to Pantridge's ward - there being no recovery room in those days.

As the number of cases of rheumatic heart disease decreased the problem of early death from coronary disease was increasing. This aspect of cardiology was to consume the rest of Pantridge's professional life and is outlined in the previous chapters of this book.

His full name was James Francis Pantridge, known to his friends and equals as Frank; to others he was JFP, or 'Frankie P' to the students and junior medical staff, though never to his face. He was endowed with a well developed Ulster sense of humour along with a rapid-fire and biting repartee. Teaching ward rounds could be intimidating with the full retinue of attendants around the bed: JFP, Sister (Head Nurse), senior and junior resident, houseman (intern), two clinical clerks (live-in medical students) and other medical students, there for the bedside clinical teaching. In the 1960s rheumatic heart disease was still common among the population. Diagnosis of the type of valvular lesion (mitral stenosis, aortic incompetence etc.) was made primarily by auscultation, and the acquisition of this clinical skill was essential. Thus, much time on teaching rounds was spent testing the students' ability in this area. If one missed the diagnosis JFP might say: *'Sister, arrange for this man to have an urgent audiogram, and perhaps an EEG would also be helpful.'* It was always risky to venture a diagnosis of aortic incompetence; if wrong, he might seize the opportunity to declare *'There is certainly incompetence here, but not of the aortic valve.'* If the answer was really bad the comment could be *'Please tell me you are a student from the Faculty of Engineering who has wandered in here by mistake.'* An incorrect answer might be followed by his careful scrutiny of the student's stethoscope and the conclusion: *'The problem lies between the ears, not with your stethoscope.'* During rounds he would make a point by poking you in the sternum with his index finger or, more emphatically, with stem of his pipe. In the modern humourless, victim-sensitive environment of medical teaching this behavior would be grounds for reprimand or worse. However, we did not feel belittled or humiliated by his humorous critique and indeed, he accepted a degree (a limited degree) of back-and-forth banter in this vein. As a result we spent much time seeking the elusive opening snap and rumbling diastolic murmur of mitral stenosis, or the soft early diastolic murmur of aortic regurgitation. On one occasion we managed to hobble a particularly annoying hyper-studious and pushy fellow student by surreptitiously stuffing cotton wool in the earpieces of his stethoscope.

At heart, Frankie P was an intensely shy man who never spoke of his experience in Singapore – or perhaps only to a few veteran classmates. We were all aware of his war record, but not of the horrific details until his autobiography was published after his retirement. It is not uncommon for war veterans to remain mute on their experiences for decades and open up in their later years. We knew that you did not drive a Japanese car if you wanted to work on his unit. As most of us did not own a car this was not a problem.

The phrase *'he did not suffer fools gladly'* is over used but undoubtedly applied to JFP; in fact, he did not even suffer people who were not fools if they disagreed with his viewpoint. Once he decided upon the right course, as he saw it, he was a straight from A to B man, with no diplomatic or other detours. At one international meeting during the question period following Pantridge's keynote lecture a noted cardiologist, known to disagree with him, spoke for some time stating his opposing view. From the podium, after a short pause, Pantridge replied *'Rubbish – next question.'*

His impatience and unwillingness to accept obstacles put in his path are exemplified by the story, apocryphal perhaps, of one golfing episode.

186

Pantridge played golf rarely and poorly. On one round his ball strayed from the fairway and came to rest behind a gorse bush, obstructing his direct route to the hole. It was during a dry hot spell and the gorse bush was parched. Using a newspaper from his golf bag and matches that accompanied his ever-present pipe he set fire to the bush and drove his ball through the ashes.

Frank Pantridge retired in 1982, having reached the mandatory retirement age for the National Health Service (NHS). As the value of his work came to be recognised around the world he continued to be honoured – particularly in the United States. This was in contrast to the slow acceptance in Britain, where the initial response varied from indifference to hostility. It was to be fifteen years after the report from Belfast before the UK Department of Health endorsed and funded the principle of pre-hospital coronary care put forward by Pantridge and Geddes. In Northern Ireland, not all of his colleagues accepted the necessity of pre-hospital coronary care, particularly if it had an impact on funding for other departments. As always, there was an element of spite and envy toward those who achieve a high profile – confirming the old adage that those who get things done annoy those who don't. That said, he could be demanding, abrasive and obnoxious in pursuit of his goals. His past experience of incompetent military and government rulers, along with his innate distrust of authority led him to treat with scathing disdain those in hospital administration who tried to block his path. He was contemptuous of the expanding lay administration within the NHS.

Pantridge's work was acknowledged by the award of CBE from the Queen in 1978. Many felt he deserved greater recognition, given the scope of his achievements in comparison to those who received higher honours because of their political and/or financial connections. He was apparently viewed as too 'controversial.' His achievements were ultimately celebrated in Ulster, more by the lay public than the medical establishment – with whom he frequently clashed. His ability to raise funds from the public to support his cardiac endeavours was legendary. He was to receive honorary degrees from Queen's University and the New University of Ulster. He was appointed to a personal professorial chair in Cardiology in the early 1970s.

In June 2009 an International Symposium to honour Frank Pantridge's legacy was held at the Queen's University of Belfast. At this meeting a portrait of JFP, commissioned in 2008, was unveiled and accepted by the university; it hangs in the Great Hall. In a lecture at that symposium, Richard Crampton, Professor of Cardiology at Charlottesville, Virginia stated: *'We now declare the obvious. Frank became and remains the undisputed champion*

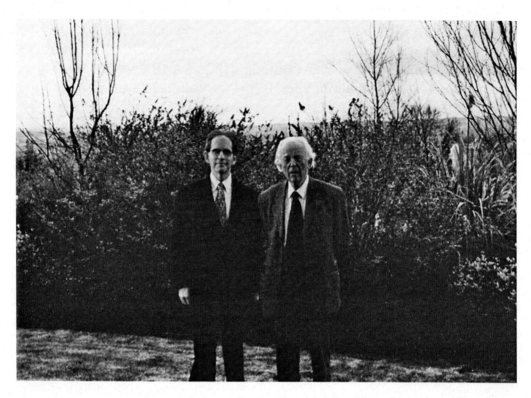

Figure 11.5 John Geddes and Frank Pantridge, Hillsborough, 2002.

of the North American Revolution in emergency care.' Earlier, in the record of the House of Representatives at the Ninety-second United States Congress it was noted: *'If Professor J. Frank Pantridge and his group at the Royal Victoria Hospital, Belfast, had not initiated the sequence of events they did in 1966, we might all still be largely ignorant of the all-important early minutes after the onset of an acute heart attack. Worse yet, we would probably still not know how little we knew.'*

Pantridge was loyal to those who worked with him, as opposed to those who did not – there were few, if any, grey areas in his appraisal. Actual praise was rare – the best you could expect was *'Look after yourself, good men are scarce.'* He did however acknowledge the sustained and indispensible contribution of John Geddes. Writing in his autobiography on the development of pre-hospital coronary care at the RVH he stated *'These might not have come about if Dr John Geddes, now in Canada alas, had not been in the cardiac department of the RVH from 1964 to 1987.'* Coming from Frank Pantridge, this was the verbal equivalent of a standing ovation. Geddes visited JFP each time he returned to Ireland (Figure 11.5). On one of these visits, towards the end of his life Pantridge quipped. *'I'm in the departure lounge but they haven't called my flight yet.'* The last scientific meeting that Pantridge and Geddes attended together was the Second Latin American Congress on Pre-hospital Coronary Care held in September 1999 in Montevideo, Uruguay. In his 84th year JFP gave a masterful keynote address and was honoured at a private luncheon with the President of Uruguay. Later they visited the small Anglican Cathedral overlooking the River Plate, in which wall plaques commemorate the sailors of the Second World War Royal Naval warships – Achilles, Ajax and Exeter. JFP was asked if he believed in God; he replied *'Well, I'm keeping my options open'.*

As he became frail JFP was admitted to a long-term care unit in the RVH. John Geddes and his wife, Florence, a former staff nurse on Wards 5 and 6, visited JFP in the unit in September 2004, about three months before his death. Pantridge produced a bottle of Scotch from his bedside locker and the ward sister provided three appropriate glasses for a resuscitative dram – even when old and frail the rules did not apply to JFP. This was the last meeting of the Pantridge-Geddes duo responsible for conceiving and developing the principles of pre-hospital coronary care.

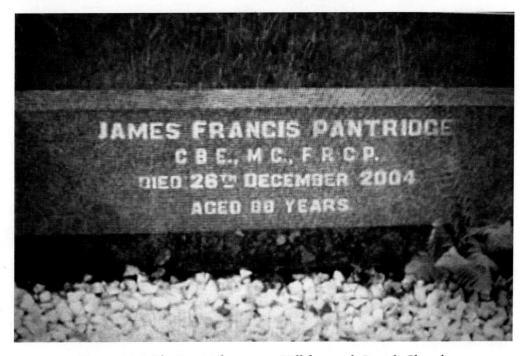

Figure 11.6 The Pantridge grave, Hillsborough Parish Church.

Frank Pantridge died in his sleep on 26th December 2004. He was buried in the family plot at Hillsborough Parish Church (Figure 11.6).

189

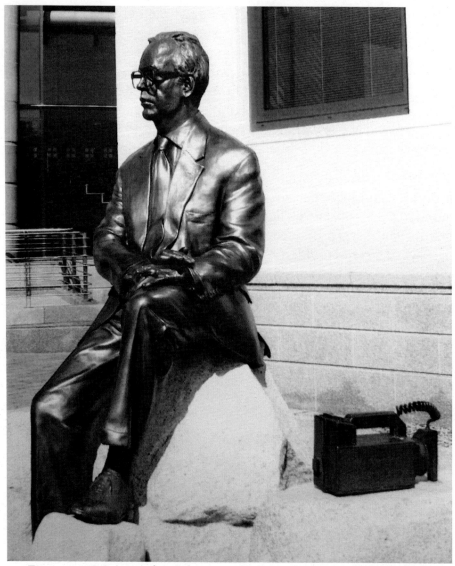

Figure 11.7 Statue of Frank Pantridge in Lisburn, Northern Ireland

He had been made a Freeman of Lisburn, and after his death the town commissioned and erected a memorial and statue (Figure 11.7). On the granite base are inscribed the words of the sign that used to hang on the wall of JFP's hospital office:

People can be divided into three groups:
Those who make things happen
Those who watch things happen and
Those who wonder what happened

No one doubted into which group Frank Pantridge fell.

Bibliography

- Barry J. Hillsborough: A Parish in the Ulster Plantation. 3rd edition. Belfast: William Mullan & Son Ltd; 1982.
- Baskett PJF. Citation for J. Frank Pantridge MC, CBE, MD, FRCP. for honorary membership of the European Resuscitation Council. Resuscitation 1994;28:183-4.
- Baskett TF, Baskett PJF. Frank Pantridge and mobile coronary care. Resuscitation 2001;48:99-104.
- Baskett PJF, Baskett TF. Frank Pantridge, 1916-2004 (obituary). Resuscitation 2005;65:7-9.
- Clarke R. The Royal Victoria Hospital, Belfast: A History 1797-1997. Belfast: Blackstaff Press; 1997.
- Geddes JS (ed). The Management of the Acute Coronary Attack: The J. Frank Pantridge Festschrift. London: Academic Press; 1986.
- Marshall R. The Royal Victoria Hospital, Belfast. 1903-1953. Belfast: WG Baird Ltd; 1953.
- McGlynn JF. British prisoners' death camp odyssey. Military History. October 2001. p30-36.
- Morrison PJ, Evans AE, Crampton RS, Julian D. Frank Pantridge's legacy: A symposium. Ulster Med J 2010;79(suppl):1-11.
- Pantridge JF. Beriberi: etiological and clinical considerations. Ulster Med J 1946;15:180-8.
- Pantridge JF, Smiley TB, Henry EW. The assessment of cases for mitral valvotomy and the results of operation. Ulster Med J 1953;22:126-37.
- Pantridge JF. An Unquiet Life: Memoirs of a Physician and Cardiologist. Antrim: Greystone Books; 1989.
- Walker G. The man who gave the world heart. Belfast Telegraph. 10 March 2001.p9.
- Obituary. BMJ 2005;330:793.

Index